Health Technical Memorandum 2010

Part 3: Validation and verification

Sterilization

London: HMSO

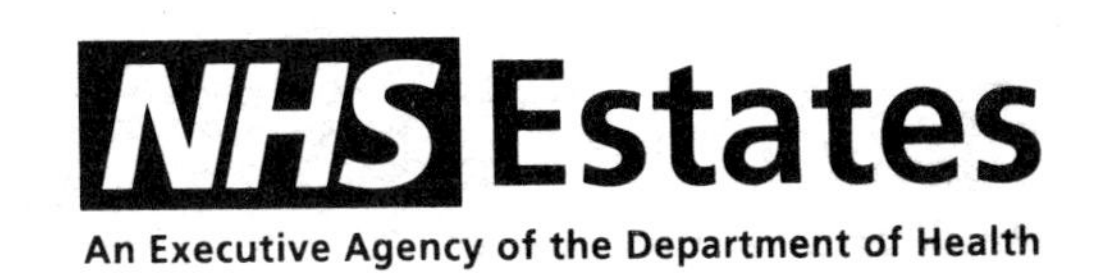

First published 1994

ISBN 0 11 321746 3

HMSO
Standing order service

Placing a standing order with HMSO BOOKS enables a customer to receive future titles in this series automatically as published. This saves the time, trouble and expense of placing individual orders and avoids the problem of knowing when to do so. For details please write to HMSO BOOKS (PC 13A/1), Publications Centre, PO Box 276, London SW8 5DT quoting reference 14.02.017. The standing order service also enables customers to receive automatically as published all material of their choice which additionally saves extensive catalogue research. The scope and selectivity of the service has been extended by new techniques, and there are more than 3,500 classifications to choose from. A special leaflet describing the service in detail may be obtained on request.

About this publication

Health Technical Memoranda (HTMs) give comprehensive advice and guidance on the design, installation and operation of specialised building and engineering technology used in the delivery of healthcare.

They are applicable to new and existing sites, and are for use at various stages during the inception, design, construction, refurbishment and maintenance of a building.

Health Technical Memorandum 2010

HTM 2010 is being published in five parts:

- Part 1 – **Management policy** – is a summary of the information required by non-technical personnel responsible for the management of sterilization services. It discusses the various types of sterilizer, for both clinical and laboratory use, and also contains guidance on legal and policy matters, and on the appointment and responsibilities of personnel. It should be read by anyone consulting this memorandum for the first time;
- Part 2 – **Design considerations** – contains information relevant to the specification and installation of new sterilizing equipment. It discusses the requirements for each type of sterilizer and outlines the specifications to be included in any contract. Practical considerations for the installation of sterilizers are discussed, including siting, heat emission, ventilation, noise and vibration, and mains services with an emphasis on steam quality;
- Part 3 – **Validation and verification** – covers all aspects of validation and periodic testing of sterilizers. It includes detailed schedules and procedures for tests and checks to be carried out for commissioning and performance qualification, and for subsequent periodic testing;
- Part 4 – **Operational management** – covers all aspects of the routine operation and maintenance of sterilizers, stressing the need for a planned maintenance programme along with the type of records to be kept. Advice on the safe and efficient operation of sterilizers is given, as

well as procedures for reporting defects and accidents;

- Part 5 – **Good practice guide** – provides advice on the fatigue life of pressure vessels, operational procedures guidance on the control of strategies, and use of the supplementary publications (log books etc). It also includes a comprehensive bibliography.

The contents of this HTM in terms of management policy and operational policy are endorsed by:

a. the Welsh Office for the NHS in Wales;

b. the Health and Personal Social Services Management Executive in Northern Ireland;

c. the National Health Service in Scotland Management Executive.

References to legislation appearing in the main text of this guidance apply to the United Kingdom as a whole, except where marginal notes indicate variations for Scotland or Northern Ireland. Where appropriate, marginal notes are also used to amplify the text.

Contents

Preface

HTM 2010 gives guidance on the choice, specification, purchase, installation, validation, periodic testing, operation and maintenance of the following types of sterilizer in use in the National Health Service:

a. clinical sterilizers:

(i) high-temperature steam sterilizers used for processing porous loads (including instruments and utensils wrapped in porous materials);

(ii) high-temperature steam sterilizers used for processing aqueous fluids in sealed containers;

(iii) high-temperature steam sterilizers used for processing unwrapped solid instruments and utensils;

(iv) dry-heat sterilizers (hot-air sterilizers);

In Scotland, LTSF sterilizers are considered to be disinfectors.

(v) low-temperature steam (LTS) disinfectors and low-temperature steam and formaldehyde (LTSF) sterilizers;

(vi) ethylene oxide (EO) sterilizers;

b. laboratory sterilizers:

(i) high-temperature steam sterilizers used with one or more specialised operating cycles;

(ii) culture media preparators.

Sterilization by irradiation is not covered.

This HTM is intended primarily as a guide for technical personnel, whether specialists in sterilizers and sterilization procedures or those responsible for maintenance and testing. It is also intended for those responsible for the day-to-day running of sterilizers, and will also be of interest to supplies officers, architects, estates managers and others in both the public and private sectors.

Scottish Health Planning Note 13, 'Sterile services department', applies in Scotland.

Detailed information on the planning and design of a sterile services department, including the level of provision of sterilizers, is given in Health Building Note 13 – 'Sterile services department'. Guidance for laboratory installations can be found in Health Building Note 15 – 'Accommodation for pathology services'.

Although this edition of HTM 2010 reflects established sterilizer technology, it is recognized that considerable scope exists for the utilisation of emerging technology in the management of sterilizers. This will be kept under review with the aim of introducing recommendations for such technology at the earliest opportunity so that the procedures essential for the efficient, safe and effective operation of sterilizers can be optimised.

Most of the British Standards for sterilizers which were applicable at the time of the last edition of this HTM, in 1980, have been either withdrawn or radically revised. Some of them, in turn, are now being replaced by European Standards which will be published during the currency of this edition of HTM 2010. Some of these European Standards support new European Union (EU) Directives on medical devices which will have a major impact on sterilization. Where practicable the information in this HTM has been aligned with existing or anticipated standards, and advice is offered where no standard has yet been formulated.

The sterilizers described in this HTM may not be suitable, without modification, for safely processing articles infected with Hazard Group 4 pathogens nor agents, such as those associated with transmissible spongiform encephalopathies, which are unusually resistant to sterilization. Design considerations for sterilizers intended to process articles infected with such organisms are discussed in Part 2.

Information about Hazard Groups may be found in the HSC document 'Categorisation of pathogens according to hazard and categories of containment' (second edition, 1990) compiled by the Advisory Committee on Dangerous Pathogens.

1.0 Introduction

General

1.1 This part of HTM 2010 covers the validation and periodic testing of the various sterilization processes used in hospitals, laboratories and other healthcare facilities.

1.2 Terminology used in sterilization has long been inconsistent and occasionally ambiguous. This HTM introduces a set of terms consistent with new European Standards (see paragraph 1.4) which, it is hoped, will in time be adopted by sterilization workers in the NHS. The Glossary contains definitions referred to in this part. A fuller list of terms will be found in Part 5, 'Good practice guide'.

1.3 The Bibliography contains full references for all the documents referred to in this part and for selected documents of which the reader should be aware. A fuller list of references relevant to sterilization will be found in Part 5.

European Standards

1.4 Part 1 of this HTM discusses the three European Union Directives on the manufacture and supply of medical devices, active implantable medical devices and in-vitro diagnostic medical devices, which are being implemented in the UK in stages from 1993 onwards. The Directives do not cover sterilization of medicinal products, as this is governed by other legislation (see Part 1).

1.5 To support the Directives, the European Committee for Standardisation (Comité Européen de Normalisation, CEN) has prepared draft European Standards on operational procedures for different methods of sterilization of medical devices. Compliance with the relevant standard is considered to be a legal presumption of compliance with the sterilization requirements of the Directive it supports. The standards require that persons responsible for sterilization operate a quality system and that part of that system is validation and routine testing of the process.

1.6 The following European Standards on the validation and routine control of sterilization processes are relevant to this part of HTM 2010:

a. EN 550 covers ethylene oxide sterilization;

b. EN 554 covers all "moist heat" sterilization. This includes porous load and fluid sterilizers (except where used for medicinal products), and sterilizers for unwrapped instruments and utensils;

c. EN 556 sets out the requirements for medical devices to be labelled "sterile".

1.7 There are no European Standards, as yet, on the use of dry-heat sterilizers, low-temperature steam disinfectors, low-temperature steam and formaldehyde sterilizers or laboratory sterilizers. A complete list of European Standards specific to sterilization is given in the Bibliography.

1.8 This edition of HTM 2010 has been written while the new standards are in the course of development. While the guidance given here is designed to be broadly consistent with the emerging standards, HTM 2010 should not be regarded as a substitute for the standards themselves when ascertaining compliance with EU Directives or the UK Regulations that implement them.

Personnel

1.9 The following personnel are referred to in this part of HTM 2010. Further information, including qualifications and areas of responsibility, can be found in Part 1.

1.10 **Management** is defined as the owner, occupier, employer, general manager, chief executive or other person of similar authority who is ultimately accountable for the sole operation of the premises.

1.11 Depending on the nature of the organisation, this role may be filled by the general manager, chief executive, laboratory director or other person of similar authority. In small, autonomous installations the user may take on this function.

1.12 The **user** is defined as the person designated by the executive manager to be responsible for the management of the sterilizer.

1.13 In a hospital the user could be a sterile services department manager, laboratory manager or theatre manager; in primary care he or she could be a general practitioner, dentist, or other health professional. Where a sterilizer is used to process medicinal products, the user is normally the production manager (see paragraph 1.20) in charge of the entire manufacturing process.

1.14 The **competent person (pressure vessels)** is defined as a person or organisation designated by management to exercise certain legal responsibilities with regard to the written scheme of examination of any pressure vessel associated with a sterilizer described in the Pressure Systems and Transportable Gas Containers Regulations 1989 (see Part 1). The shorter term "competent person" is used in this HTM.

The Pressure Systems and Transportable Gas Containers Regulations (Northern Ireland) 1991 apply in Northern Ireland.

1.15 The **authorised person (sterilizers)** is defined as a person designated by management to provide independent auditing and advice on sterilizers and sterilization and to review and witness documentation on validation. The shorter term "authorised person" is used in this HTM.

1.16 A list of suitably qualified authorised persons (sterilizers) is maintained by the Institution of Hospital Engineering (see Appendix 1).

1.17 The **test person (sterilizers)** is defined as a person designated by the executive manager to carry out validation and periodic testing of sterilizers. The shorter term "test person" is used in this HTM.

1.18 The **maintenance person (sterilizers)** is defined as a person designated by the executive manager to carry out maintenance duties on sterilizers. The shorter term "maintenance person" is used in this HTM.

1.19 The **microbiologist (sterilizers)** is defined as a person designated by the executive manager to be responsible for advising the user on microbiological aspects of the sterilization of non-medicinal products. The shorter term "microbiologist" is used in this HTM.

1.20 The **production manager** is defined as a person designated by the executive manager to be responsible for the production of medicinal products.

1.21 The **quality controller** is defined as a person designated by the executive manager to be responsible for quality control of medicinal products with authority to establish, verify and implement all quality control and quality assurance procedures.

1.22 The **laboratory safety officer** is defined as a person designated by the executive manager to be responsible for all aspects of laboratory safety including equipment, personnel and training relating to safety issues, and ensuring compliance with safety legislation and guidelines.

1.23 An **operator** is defined as any person with the authority to operate a sterilizer, including the noting of sterilizer instrument readings and simple housekeeping duties.

1.24 The **manufacturer** is defined as a person or organisation responsible for the manufacture of a sterilizer.

1.25 The **contractor** is defined as a person or organisation designated by the executive manager to be responsible for the supply and installation of the sterilizer, and for the conduct of the installation checks and tests. The contractor is commonly the manufacturer of the sterilizer.

Safety

1.26 Extensive guidance on the safe operation of the various types of sterilizer is given in Part 4, 'Operational management'. As far as testing is concerned, normal safety precautions are adequate except in the case of sterilizers used to process infectious materials, and sterilizers using gaseous sterilants, as described below. Users are recommended to operate a permit-to-work system to ensure that such sterilizers are declared safe to work on, and that personnel working on them have documented authority to do so.

Infectious materials

1.27 All sterilizers have the potential to process infectious materials, but attention is drawn to certain laboratory sterilizers with cycles expressly designed for the routine making-safe of discard material that is or may be contaminated with pathogenic micro-organisms. Note also that laboratory sterilizers without a make-safe cycle may be occasionally used to process infected material in the event of the designated machine being out of service. The user should therefore ensure that personnel working on laboratory sterilizers wear appropriate protective clothing and are fully informed of any hazards that may be present. Further guidance may be found in the HSC document 'Safe working and the prevention of infection in clinical laboratories: model rules for staff and visitors', compiled by the Health Services Advisory Committee.

Gaseous sterilants

The Control of Substances Hazardous to Health Regulations (Northern Ireland) 1990 apply in Northern Ireland.

1.28 Low-temperature steam and formaldehyde (LTSF) sterilizers and ethylene oxide (EO) sterilizers both use toxic gases in the sterilization process. Occupational exposure to formaldehyde and EO is controlled by the Control of Substances Hazardous to Health (COSHH) Regulations (see Part 1). Maximum exposure limits are set out in the annual Guidance Note EH40, 'Occupational exposure limits', published by the Health and Safety Executive (HSE) (see Bibliography). At the time of writing (1994) the limits are as shown in Table 1. These limits are statutory maxima but should not be regarded as representing a safe working exposure; employers have a legal obligation to ensure that the level of exposure is reduced so far as is reasonably practicable and in any case below the maximum exposure limit.

Gas	Short-term exposure limit [ppm]	[mg m-3]	Long-term exposure limit [ppm]	[mg m-3]
Formaldehyde	2	2.5	2	2.5
Ethylene oxide	15	30.0	5	10.0

The short-term exposure limit (STEL) is the average exposure over any 15-minute period.

The long-term exposure limit (LTEL) is the exposure over any 24-hour period expressed as a single uniform exposure over an 8-hour period.

COSHH does not specify a STEL for EO. In such cases the STEL is deemed to be three times the LTEL in accordance with the recommendations of the Health and Safety Executive.

(Source: HSE Guidance Note EH40 (1994))

Table 1 Maximum exposure limits for atmospheric formaldehyde and ethylene oxide

1.29 Certain tests in this document require that the sterilant gases be replaced with a suitable non-hazardous substitute:

a. for LTSF sterilizers, the primary material for generating formaldehyde (usually formalin) should be replaced with water;

b. for EO sterilizers where the gas is supplied from cylinders, the sterilant gas should be replaced with a suitable non-toxic, non-flammable gas or gas mixture admitted to the chamber through the EO supply system (including the vaporiser). Air may be used if the system is known to be free of residual traces of EO sufficient to cause an explosive or fire hazard (see paragraph 6.54 for a specification for a suitable monitoring instrument), but nitrogen is recommended as being safe in all circumstances;

c. for EO sterilizers where the gas is supplied from cartridges contained within the chamber, no substitute is normally necessary because of the small amounts of EO present in the system. If a substitute is thought to be desirable, nitrogen cartridges may be used.

2.0 Testing of sterilizers

Introduction

2.1 Sterilization is a process whose efficacy cannot be verified retrospectively by inspection or testing of the product. For this reason sterilization processes have to be validated before use, the performance of the process routinely monitored, and the equipment maintained.

2.2 Means of assuring that a sterilizer is fit for its intended purpose will include tests and checks carried out during the various stages of manufacture, after delivery, during validation and periodically thereafter. Tests will also be required before a sterilizer is returned to service after modification.

2.3 The philosophy of testing and maintenance embodies three main principles to ensure that required standards of performance and safety are attained and sustained:

a. all sterilizers are subject to a planned programme of tests to monitor their performance;

b. all sterilizers are subject to a planned programme of preventive maintenance irrespective of whether or not a preventive maintenance scheme is being operated on the premises generally;

c. expertise on all aspects of the testing of sterilizers should be available at two levels; these are represented by the authorised person (sterilizers) and the test person.

2.4 The scheduled test programmes include simple procedures undertaken by the user, as well as more complex tests undertaken by the test person to demonstrate that the equipment is functioning satisfactorily.

2.5 Schedules for installation checks, validation tests and periodic tests are presented in Chapters 3, 4 and 5, and discussed below. Where appropriate, the schedules refer to detailed test procedures described in later chapters.

2.6 Maintenance of sterilizers is dealt with in Part 4 of this HTM.

Responsibilities for validation

2.7 Sterilizers should be commissioned on site using the procedures described in this HTM. The purchaser, manufacturer and contractor have distinct responsibilities.

Purchaser

2.8 Management should nominate an authorised person (sterilizers) to provide advice on validation.

2.9 The test person should witness the installation checks and tests carried out by the contractor, and arrange for test loads to be supplied as required.

2.10 The test person should carry out the commissioning tests and performance qualification tests. (Some of the performance qualification tests on LTSF and EO sterilizers are the responsibility of the user.)

Manufacturer

2.11 The manufacturer should ensure that the sterilizer is designed, manufactured and tested within a quality system such as that given in BS5750. The extent of testing will depend on whether the manufacturer has obtained a current certificate of compliance to a relevant British or European Standard by means of a type test for the particular type and size of sterilizer:

a. where a certificate is available, the manufacturer may limit the works tests to those which demonstrate compliance with the specification;

b. when a certificate is not available, such as for a one-off design, works tests should (except for the sound pressure test) include those listed as commissioning tests in Tables 2 and 3 (see Chapter 4). This option is expensive.

Contractor

2.12 The contractor (who may also be the manufacturer) should complete the installation checks and tests specified in Chapter 3 to the satisfaction of the test person before the sterilizer can be accepted for use in accordance with the contract.

2.13 The contractor should provide the test instruments and equipment (but not the test loads, see paragraph 2.9) required for the installation checks and tests, and should satisfy the authorised person that their accuracy, calibration and condition meet the requirements for test instruments specified in Chapter 6, and that the calibration of each instrument has been checked on site and is satisfactory.

The validation process

2.14 Validation is defined as a documented procedure for obtaining, recording and interpreting the results needed to show that a process will consistently yield a product complying with predetermined specifications. Validation is considered as a total process which consists of commissioning followed by performance qualification (Figure 1).

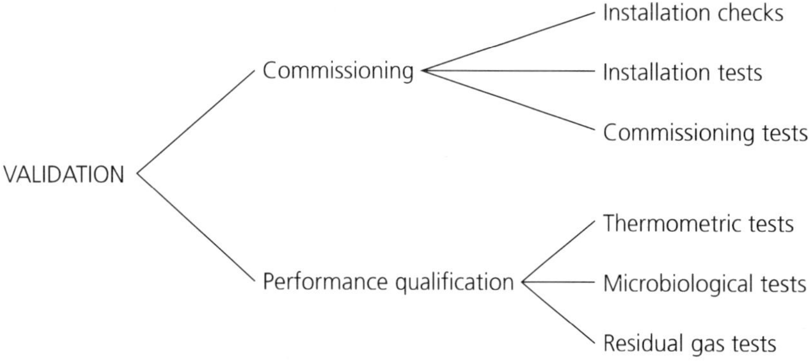

Figure 1 The validation process

Commissioning

2.15 Commissioning is defined as the process of obtaining and documenting evidence that the equipment has been provided and installed in accordance with its specifications, and that it functions within predetermined limits when operated in accordance with operational instructions.

2.16 Commissioning consists of a series of installation checks and installation tests (often identified as "installation qualification" and "equipment qualification") to be carried out by the contractor, and a series of commissioning tests to be carried out by the test person.

Installation checks

2.17 On delivery of the sterilizer, the contractor should carry out the required installation checks to establish that the sterilizer has been provided and installed correctly, is safe to operate, does not interfere with nearby equipment and that all connected services are satisfactory and do not restrict the attainment of conditions for sterilization.

2.18 Ancillary equipment, such as service supplies and ventilation systems, should be checked by the contractor responsible for their installation.

2.19 The schedule for installation checks is set out in Chapter 3.

Installation tests

2.20 When the installation checks have been completed, the contractor should carry out the required installation tests to demonstrate that the sterilizer is working satisfactorily. The contractor is not required to carry out any thermometric tests unless previously specified in the contract. Any assistance required from the department in which the sterilizer is installed should be agreed between the contractor and the purchaser.

2.21 If any maintenance or modification work is carried out on the steam, water or piped gas services after the installation tests have been completed, the tests should be repeated by the test person before the commissioning tests commence.

2.22 The schedule for installation tests is set out in Chapter 4.

Commissioning tests

2.23 When the sterilizer has been accepted, the test person should carry out a sequence of commissioning tests to evaluate basic performance and safety. Some of these commissioning tests are identical to those specified as installation tests, and need not be repeated if commissioning follows within seven days of the installation tests.

2.24 The schedule for commissioning tests is set out in Chapter 4.

Performance qualification

2.25 Performance qualification (PQ) is defined as the process of obtaining and documenting evidence that the equipment as commissioned will produce an acceptable product when operated according to process specification.

2.26 PQ consists of tests designed to show that sterilization conditions are attained throughout a production load. A thermometric test is sufficient for most sterilizers but an additional microbiological test is required for sterilizers using gaseous sterilants, and may be necessary for any sterilizer where loading conditions cannot be validated solely by thermometric methods.

2.27 In principle, a PQ test is required for each loading condition that the sterilizer is intended to process. In practice, a test on a single "reference load" may be valid for a range of less demanding loading conditions and in some cases, notably porous loads, the tests specified for commissioning will often provide sufficient evidence for performance qualification.

2.28 The schedule for performance qualification tests is set out with the commissioning tests in Chapter 4. Further information and detailed procedures for performance qualification are given in Chapter 8.

Documentation

2.29 Accurate and efficient keeping of records is an essential part of the management of a sterilizer. A recommended system, based on a plant history file and a sterilizer process log, is described in Part 4 of this HTM.

Summary sheets

2.30 On the completion of the validation process, and before leaving the premises, the test person should prepare summary sheets for the user containing the results of the commissioning and PQ tests, and essential working data. At the request of the user the test person should also supply graphical representations of cycle variables obtained from the thermometric tests. The sheets should be signed by the test person and countersigned by the user to certify that the sterilizer is fit for use. Summary sheets should be kept in the sterilizer process log for ready reference by the user. A set of model summary sheets is given in Appendix 3.

2.31 At the same time the test person should provide the user with copies of any master process records (see paragraph 8.58) required for routine production.

Validation report

2.32 Within one month of the completion of the validation process the test person should prepare a full validation report. It should include the following:

a. all the data, supplied by the contractor, collected during the installation checks specified in Chapter 3 and the installation tests specified in Chapter 4, with written confirmation from the contractor that they meet the manufacturer's specifications;

b. written confirmation from the contractor that the calibration of all instruments and gauges fitted to the sterilizer has been verified;

c. all the data collected during the commissioning tests specified in Chapter 4, with written confirmation from the test person that they meet the requirements of the tests;

d. data showing the correlation between the performance of the instruments fitted on the sterilizer and the test instruments used for commissioning and performance qualification;

e. all the data collected during the performance qualification tests in the form of PQ reports (see paragraph 8.54), with written confirmation from the test person and the user and (for medicinal products) the quality controller of the loading conditions (see paragraph 8.7) which may be satisfactorily processed in the sterilizer.

2.33 If any of the data is in the form of electronic data files, the report should include copies of disks or tapes containing the data in a format agreed with the user, and a print-out of each disk or tape directory showing clearly where the data for each test are to be found.

2.34 The test person should certify that all tests and checks have been carried out and that the results are satisfactory. The microbiologist should sign the records of any microbiological tests. The complete validation report should be examined and countersigned by the authorised person.

2.35 The validation report should be given to the user for the plant history file and a copy retained by the test person. Copies should be sent to the authorised person and, on request, to the quality controller and the microbiologist.

Periodic tests

2.36 After the validation process has been completed, and the sterilizer is passed into service, it is subject to a schedule of periodic tests at daily, weekly, quarterly and yearly intervals. These tests are the shared responsibility of the user and the test person.

2.37 The yearly test schedule is essentially a revalidation schedule. It provides for performance requalification (PRQ) tests to confirm that data collected during performance qualification remain valid.

2.38 The schedule of periodic tests is set out in Chapter 5.

Revalidation

2.39 Revalidation is the process of confirming that the operational data acquired during validation remain valid. It consists of recommissioning followed by performance requalification. Revalidation is required on the following occasions:

a. when modifications or engineering work are carried out which could affect the performance of the sterilizer, for example:
    (i) when a sterilizer is to be returned to service after the repair of a serious defect (see Part 4);
    (ii) when the inspection of a sterilizer pressure vessel by the competent person requires the removal of components which could affect the performance of the sterilizer (if the inspection immediately precedes a yearly test, recommissioning is not necessary);
    (iii) when the preset values of cycle variables have been modified;
    (iv) when the software in a computer control system has been upgraded or otherwise modified;

b. when the sterilizer is to be returned to service after investigation and correction of unacceptable deviations from performance data established during validation, for example:
    (i) when the pattern of a batch process record is outside the limits specified on the master process record;
    (ii) when the sterilizer fails a periodic test;

c. when there is a demand for revalidation by an authorized inspectorate or licensing authority;

d. whenever the user or authorised person advises that revalidation is necessary.

2.40 The revalidation procedure is identical to that prescribed for the yearly tests set out in Chapter 5.

Repeat validation

2.41 On occasions, usually rare, it will be necessary to repeat the validation procedure to obtain a new set of commissioning and performance qualification data to replace the set originally obtained during validation. Repeat validation is required on the following occasions:

a. when the sterilizer is subject to modifications of such a nature that the validation data must be presumed to be no longer valid, for example:
   (i) when a sterilizer, other than a transportable, has been moved and installed at a new site;
   (ii) when a sterilizer has been dismantled or extensively overhauled or modified;
   (iii) when a new operating cycle has been introduced;

b. when revalidation or a yearly test fails to confirm the validity of the original validation data and no obvious cause can be found;

c. whenever the authorised person advises that repeat validation is necessary;

d. when there is a demand for repeat validation by an authorised inspectorate or licensing authority.

2.42 The authorised person should advise on which elements of the validation process need be repeated. For example, it will not be necessary to repeat all of the installation checks.

Types of test

2.43 Although many tests are listed in the schedules, they fall into a few basic categories as follows.

2.44 **Automatic control tests** are designed to show that the operating cycle functions correctly as evidenced by the values of the cycle variables indicated and recorded by the instruments fitted permanently to the sterilizer.

2.45 **Thermometric tests** use accurate measuring equipment to monitor temperatures and pressures independently of the instruments fitted to the sterilizer. They provide the assurance that the temperature requirements for sterilization are met:

a. thermometric tests for a **small load** are designed for two purposes. In sterilizers with an active air removal system they demonstrate that the sterilizer is capable of removing air from a small load in which air from a near-empty chamber has been retained. In cycles for fluid loads they demonstrate that sufficient condensate will be collected for cooling purposes, and that the initial temperature overshoot is kept within acceptable limits;

b. thermometric tests for a **full load** are designed to show that sterilization conditions are present in a test load of specified maximum mass and of sufficient size to fill the usable chamber space. In certain circumstances they may also serve as PQ tests for loading conditions which present a lesser challenge to the operating cycle than the specified full load (see paragraph 8.7).

2.46 **Microbiological tests** are designed to show that sterilization conditions are attained where thermometric methods are inadequate, that is, for LTSF and EO sterilizers and for exceptional loading conditions in other sterilizers.

2.47 Other tests, specific to certain types of sterilizer, are designed to show that the steam supply is suitable, the sterilizer does not produce too much noise, the chamber is airtight, gaseous sterilants are not released into the environment, and safety devices are functioning correctly.

Procedure on failure of a test

2.48 A correctly installed and maintained sterilizer should have no difficulty in complying with either the validation tests or the periodic tests. As a rule, a failure of a test implies that the sterilizer is not working to specification, and it should be withdrawn from service and the failure investigated. In practice the immediate action to be taken is a matter for judgement based on the nature of the failure and experience gained in using the sterilizer. In some cases it may be acceptable for the sterilizer to continue in service under restricted operating conditions until the failure can be investigated. The authorised person and the user should agree in advance on how to handle test failures.

2.49 It should be emphasised that the user has the ultimate responsibility for certifying that the sterilizer is fit for use.

3.0 Schedule of installation checks

Introduction

3.1 On delivery of the sterilizer the contractor should carry out the installation checks set out in this chapter and included in the contract to establish that the sterilizer has been provided and installed correctly, is safe to operate, does not interfere with other equipment and that all connected services are satisfactory and do not restrict the attainment of conditions for sterilization.

3.2 Installation checks on services and other ancillary equipment should be carried out by the contractor responsible for their installation. These checks should be completed satisfactorily before starting the checks on the sterilizer itself.

3.3 Any checks specified here which are not included in the contract should be completed by the test person before commissioning begins.

3.4 As a safety precaution, checks on LTSF sterilizers should be carried out on the LTS cycle only. Checks on EO sterilizers should be carried out using a non-hazardous substitute for the sterilant as described in Chapter 1.

Checks on ancillary equipment

3.5 Ancillary equipment should ideally be installed and commissioned before the validation procedure for the sterilizer begins. Where the checks require the sterilizer to be operating, the test person should carry them out in cooperation with the sterilizer contractor. The sterilizer contractor is not responsible for the correct functioning of services and other ancillary equipment unless agreed in the contract.

Engineering services

3.6 Check that the following requirements are met:

a. the engineering services are installed correctly, they are adequate to meet the demands of the sterilizer, and they do not leak;

b. drains remove effluent effectively when all plant in the vicinity, including the sterilizer, is connected and operating;

c. the water economy system (if fitted) operates correctly;

d. for EO sterilizers supplied from cylinders, the system complies with the requirements of Part 2, and all gas lines are free of leaks.

Additional checks for LTSF and EO sterilizers

3.7 LTSF and EO sterilizers require further checks to the ventilation and safety systems because of the use of toxic gases.

3.8 For both LTSF and EO, check that the ventilation systems within the loading area, plantroom and manifold room meet the requirements of Part 2. Pay particular attention to the following:

a. they meet the manufacturer's specification;

b. air flow is from the operator towards the sterilizer, and air does not flow from the plantroom into the loading area;

c. exhaust systems are non-recirculating and their discharges comply with safety regulations;

d. if the air flow is insufficient to cause a minimum of 10 air changes an hour:

   (i) a warning is given;

   (ii) the door cannot be opened at the end of the operating cycle;

   (iii) a new cycle cannot be started.

3.9 Check that the local exhaust ventilation system meets the requirements of Part 2. Pay particular attention to the following:

a. air flow is from the operator towards the sterilizer, and air does not flow from the plantroom into the loading area;

b. the rate of flow complies with that specified in Part 2;

c. the exhaust discharge complies with safety regulations specified in Part 2.

3.10 Check that the drain from the sterilizer to the drainage system is trapped, sealed and vented to a safe position, as described in Part 2.

Additional checks for EO sterilizers

3.11 Check that the local exhaust ventilation system meets the following requirements in addition to those in paragraph 3.9:

a. manual control switches are located in prominent, easily accessible positions, such as in the EO cylinder change area;

b. the system operates whenever any one of the manual switches is operated;

c. it operates automatically at the end of an operating cycle and before the door is opened;

d. it operates whenever any of the gas detectors sense that the atmospheric concentration of EO exceeds the short-term exposure limit specified in Table 1.

3.12 Check that EO safety installations meet the requirements of Part 2. Pay particular attention to the following:

a. notices concerning emergency procedures, safety and restricted access are displayed in prominent positions;

b. where gas is supplied from cylinders:

   (i) environmental alarm and emergency systems are installed and operate in accordance with the specification;

   (ii) emergency protective equipment is provided and stored in designated areas.

Checks on the sterilizer

3.13 The following checks presume that engineering services and other ancillary equipment are functioning correctly.

Preliminary checks

3.14 After the sterilizer has been installed, check that the following requirements are met:

a. the manufacturer has supplied all the documents specified in the contract;

b. the sterilizer has been supplied and installed in accordance with the contract;

c. calibration verification certificates for the temperature and pressure instruments and controllers are supplied;

d. no defects are apparent from a visual inspection of the sterilizer;

e. all supports, bases and fixings are secure and without imposed strain from service connections;

f. thermal insulation is in good condition and securely attached;

g. security and settings of door safety switches and door-locking components are in compliance with data provided by the manufacturer;

h. keys, codes or tools required to operate locked controls are supplied and operate satisfactorily. Each key, code or tool unlocks only the control for which it is intended, and cannot unlock controls on other sterilizers in the vicinity;

j. loading trolleys and other aids are effective and safe in use.

3.15 Check that the electrical equipment on the sterilizer is correctly connected to the electrical service. Carry out the following electrical tests:

a. insulation resistance;

b. phase sequence (for three-phase installations);

c. polarity;

d. bonding and earth continuity;

e. emergency stop.

Functional checks

3.16 During an operating cycle with an empty chamber, check that the following requirements are met (several cycles may be necessary to complete all the checks):

a. the selection of automatic or manual control is by key, code or tool. When the controller is in manual mode, the automatic control is inactivated. When the controller is in automatic mode, the manual control is inactivated;

b. under automatic control, steam, compressed air, formaldehyde or EO cannot be admitted into the chamber, and the operating cycle cannot start, until the door is locked and sealed. Under manual control, the operator can advance the cycle only sequentially through each stage. Any stages designed to remove formaldehyde or EO from the chamber and load cannot be circumvented;

c. throughout the cycle, indicated and recorded steam, water, air and gas pressures are within the limits specified by the manufacturer;

d. throughout the cycle, there are no leaks of steam, water, air, gas or effluent;

e. there is no evidence of interference to or from other equipment connected to the same services;

f. there is no evidence of electromagnetic interference to or from other equipment;

g. operation and readings of all instruments appear satisfactory, including return to zero (this may not be achievable with combined pressure and vacuum gauges);

h. the temperature of surfaces routinely handled by the operator does not exceed that specified in Part 2;

j. the effluent temperature does not exceed that specified in Part 2.

3.17 At the end of a cycle check that the following requirements are met:

a. the door opening system cannot be operated until the chamber vent valve is open, and the chamber pressure is within 200 mbar of atmospheric;

b. door retaining parts cannot be released until the seal between the door and chamber has been broken, and the chamber is effectively vented to atmospheric pressure;

c. the door interlock system is either fail-safe or is fitted with at least two independent interlocks. Failure of one interlock, or any one service, does not allow the door to be opened when conditions within the chamber would cause a hazard, for example, pressure in excess of 200 mbar, unacceptable level of sterilant gas, or temperature of fluid in sealed containers above 80°C (glass) or 90°C (plastic);

d. for EO sterilizers, the operating cycle automatically returns to either the gas removal stage or the flushing stage if the door has remained sealed for more than 15 minutes after the admission of air;

e. the automatic controller has operated in accordance with the specification.

Response to external faults

3.18 It is necessary to check that the sterilizer reacts correctly and safely when exposed to a number of external fault conditions, that is, a safety hazard is not created and a false indication of "cycle complete" is not obtained. During each stage of an operating cycle, check the response of the sterilizer to the following simulated faults (where appropriate to the type of sterilizer):

a. operation of the emergency stop button;

b. power failure;

c. steam pressure too low;

d. steam pressure too high;

e. water pressure too low;

f. compressed air pressure too low;

g. failure of sterilant gas supply (LTSF and EO);

j. failure of room ventilation (LTSF and EO).

4.0 Schedule of validation tests

Introduction

4.1 Installation tests are carried out by the contractor to demonstrate compliance with specifications, and may be repeated by the test person if required. Commissioning and performance qualification tests are carried out by the test person.

4.2 The schedules for the tests are set out for each type of clinical sterilizer in Table 2 and for laboratory sterilizers in Table 3. Each test is cross-referenced to a detailed description of the test procedure in a later chapter. The tests should be carried out with the sterilizer at normal working temperature (a warming-up cycle may be needed) and completed in the order shown.

4.3 The laboratory machine known as a Köch steamer is not listed here. Where it is used primarily for melting agar, validation tests are not required. Where it is to be used for the disinfection of a product, the thermometric tests prescribed in Table 3b for the culture media cycle should be followed.

4.4 The calibration of thermometric test equipment should be checked before and after the thermometric tests as described in paragraphs 6.32–39.

4.5 In principle, performance qualification tests should be carried out after the commissioning tests have been completed. However, for sterilizers with an active air removal system, thermometric PQ tests may be performed while the sensors used in the commissioning tests are still in place and before any final vacuum leak test. This is provided for in the schedules. Where tests on EO sterilizers require EO gas to be in the chamber, however, sensors should either be removed from the chamber or else disconnected from the recorder and the wires grounded to the body of the sterilizer (see note (d) to Table 2f).

4.6 Chapter 8 describes general procedures for conducting performance qualification tests and generating master process records.

Table 2 Schedule of validation tests for clinical sterilizers

		Ref
	Installation tests – contractor	
1.	Vacuum leak test	11.2
2.	Verification of calibration of sterilizer instruments	6.32
3.	Automatic control test	12.1
	Commissioning tests – test person	
1.	Steam non-condensable gas test	9.4
2.	Steam superheat test	9.20
3.	Steam dryness test	9.30
4.	Vacuum leak test	11.2
5.	Vacuum leak test (temperature and pressure sensors connected)	11.2
6.	Automatic control test	12.1
7.	Verification of calibration of sterilizer instruments*	12.2
8.	Chamber wall temperature test	13.3
9.	Air detector performance test for a small load	11.45
10.	Air detector performance test for a full load	11.53
11.	Thermometric test for a full load	13.15
12.	[Load dryness test]*	13.25
13.	Thermometric test for a small load	13.7
14.	[Load dryness test]*	13.25
15.	Thermometric test for a small load (to check consistency with test 13)	13.7
	Performance qualification tests (see below)	
16.	Vacuum leak test (sensors removed)	11.2
17.	Air detector function test	11.60
18.	Bowie-Dick test for steam penetration	13.3
19.	[Sound pressure test]	10.1
	Performance qualification tests – test person	
1.	Thermometric tests for performance qualification as required by the user[a]	8.13
2.	Hospital load dryness check	13.25

* May be done at the same time as the preceding test.

[ ] Optional test, to be done at the user's discretion.

a. Not normally required for loads processed in a sterile services department (SSD) (see paragraph 8.7).

Table 2a Validation tests for porous load sterilizers

		Ref
	Installation tests – contractor	
1.	Verification of calibration of sterilizer instruments	6.32
2.	Heat exchanger integrity test	14.4
3.	Automatic control test	12.1
	Commissioning tests – test person	
1.	Automatic control test	12.1
2.	Verification of calibration of sterilizer instruments*	12.2
3.	Chamber temperature profile	7.21
4.	Thermometric test for a small load	14.21
5.	Thermometric test for a full load	14.10
6.	Coolant quality test	14.32
7.	[Sound pressure test]	10.1
	Performance qualification tests – test person	
1.	Thermometric tests for performance qualification as required by the user and the quality controller (for medicinal products) or by the user (other loads).	8.13

* May be done at the same time as the preceding test.
[ ] Optional test, to be done at the user's discretion.

Table 2b Validation tests for fluid sterilizers

		Ref
	Installation tests – contractor[a]	
1.	Verification of calibration of sterilizer instruments	6.32
2.	Automatic control test	12.1
	Commissioning tests – test person	
1.	Automatic control test	12.1
2.	Verification of calibration of sterilizer instruments*	12.2
3.	Chamber temperature profile	7.21
4.	Chamber overheat cut-out test[b]	15.3
5.	Thermometric test for a small load	15.7
6.	Thermometric test for a full load	15.13
7.	Thermometric test for a small load (to check consistency with test 5)	15.7
8.	[Sound pressure test][a]	10.1
	Performance qualification tests – test person	
1.	Thermometric tests for performance qualification as required by the user	8.13

* May be done at the same time as the preceding test.
[ ] Optional test, to be done at the user's discretion.
a. Not required for transportable sterilizers.
b. Not required where steam is supplied from a source external to the chamber.

Table 2c Validation tests for sterilizers for unwrapped instruments and utensils

		Ref
	Installation tests – contractor	
1.	Verification of calibration of sterilizer instruments	6.32
2.	Automatic control test	16.4
	Commissioning tests – test person	
1.	Automatic control test	16.4
2.	Verification of calibration of sterilizer instruments*	12.2
3.	Chamber temperature profile	7.21
4.	Chamber overheat cut-out test	16.8
5.	Air filter integrity test	16.13
	Performance qualification tests (see below)	
6.	[Thermometric test for a full load]	16.33
	Performance qualification tests – test person	
1.	Thermometric tests for performance qualification as required by the user and quality controller (medicinal products) or by the user (other loads)	16.22

* May be done at the same time as the preceding test.

[ ] Optional test, to be done at the user's discretion. The full-load test need be done only if the sterilizer fails a PQ test.

Table 2d Validation tests for dry-heat sterilizers

		Ref
	Installation tests – contractor	
1.	Vacuum leak test	11.2
2.	Verification of calibration of sterilizer instruments	6.32
3.	Automatic control test	12.1
4.	Vacuum leak monitor test	11.19
	Commissioning tests – test person	
1.	Steam non-condensable gas test	9.4
2.	Steam superheat test	9.20
3.	Steam dryness test	9.30
4.	Vacuum leak test	11.2
5.	Vacuum leak test (temperature and pressure sensors connected)	11.2
6.	Automatic control test	12.1
7.	Verification of calibration of sterilizer instruments*	12.2
8.	Vacuum leak monitor test	11.19
9.	Chamber temperature profile	7.21
10.	Chamber overheat cut-out test	17.4
11.	Chamber wall temperature test	17.10
12.	Thermometric test for a small load	17.15
13.	[Load dryness test]*	13.25
14.	Thermometric test for a full load (LTS)	17.23
15.	Thermometric test for a small load (to check consistency with test 12)	17.15
16.	Microbiological test for basic performance (LTSF)	17.40
17.	Environmental formaldehyde vapour test (LTSF)	17.32
	Performance qualification tests (see below)	
18.	Vacuum leak test (sensors removed)	11.2
19.	[Sound pressure test]	10.1
	Performance qualification tests – test person	
1.	Thermometric tests for performance qualification as required by the user	8.13
2.	Microbiological tests for performance qualification as required by the user (LTSF)	17.50
3.	Environmental gas tests (LTSF)*	8.37
	Performance qualification tests – user	
1.	Tests for degassing time (LTSF)	8.46

* May be done at the same time as the preceding test.
[ ] Optional test, to be done at the user's discretion.

Table 2e Validation tests for LTS disinfectors and LTSF sterilizers

		Ref
	Installation tests – contractor	
1.	Verification of calibration of sterilizer instruments	6.32
2.	Vacuum leak test	11.2
3.	Pressure leak test[a]	11.24
4.	Automatic control test	12.1
	Commissioning tests – test person	
1.	Vacuum leak test	11.2
2.	Pressure leak test[a]	11.24
3.	Vacuum leak test (temperature, pressure and RH sensors connected)	11.2
4.	Pressure leak test[a]	11.24
5.	Automatic control test	12.1
6.	Verification of calibration of sterilizer instruments*	12.2
7.	Vacuum leak monitor test	11.19
8.	Chamber temperature profile	7.21
9.	Chamber overheat cut-out test	18.4
10.	Chamber space temperature test	18.11
11.	Chamber wall temperature test	18.16
12.	Gas circulation test[b,d]	
13.	Microbiological test for gas exposure time[c,d]	18.20
	Performance qualification tests (see below)	
14.	Vacuum leak test (sensors removed)	11.2
15.	Pressure leak test[a]	11.24
16.	[Sound pressure test]	10.1
	Performance qualification tests – test person	
1.	Thermometric tests for performance qualification as required by the user	18.36
2.	Microbiological tests for performance qualification as required by the user[d]	18.49
3.	Environmental gas tests*	8.37
	Performance qualification test – user	
1.	Tests for degassing time	8.46

* May be done at the same time as the preceding test.

[ ] Optional test, to be done at the user's discretion.

a. Required only where the sterilizer operates above atmospheric pressure.

b. Required only where a circulating fan is fitted. Instrumentation is used to demonstrate that pressures and flows specified by the manufacturer are obtained.

c. May be omitted if test data are provided by the manufacturer.

d. To avoid risk of sparking, tests using EO gas should not be done while temperature sensors are in the chamber. Providing safe operating procedures are not compromised, it may be acceptable to disconnect the sensors from the recorder and ground the wires to the body of the sterilizer.

Table 2f Validation tests for ethylene oxide sterilizers

Table 3 Schedule of validation tests for laboratory sterilizers

		Ref
	Installation tests – contractor	
1.	Vacuum leak test[a]	11.2
2.	Verification of calibration of sterilizer instruments	6.32
3.	Automatic control test for each operating cycle	12.1
4.	Thermal door-lock override test	19.64
	Commissioning tests – test person	
1.	Vacuum leak test[a]	11.2
2.	Vacuum leak test (temperature and pressure sensors connected)[a]	11.2
3.	Automatic control test for each operating cycle	12.1
4.	Verification of calibration of sterilizer instruments*	12.2
5.	Chamber temperature profile	7.21
6.	Tests for make-safe of small plastic discard	
	(i) Thermometric test for a small load	19.16
	(ii) Thermometric test for a full load	19.7
7.	Tests for make-safe of contained fluid discard	
	(i) Thermometric test for a small load	19.37
	(ii) Thermometric test for a full load	19.24
8.	Tests for sterilization of culture media	
	(i) Thermometric test for a small load	19.37
	(ii) Thermometric test for a full load	19.24
9.	Tests for disinfection of fabrics	
	(i) Thermometric test for a small load	13.7
10.	Tests for sterilization of glassware and equipment	
	(i) Thermometric test for a small load	19.61
	(ii) Thermometric test for a full load	19.52
11.	Tests for free steaming	
	(i) Thermometric test for a full load	19.24
	Performance qualification tests (see below)[b]	
12.	Vacuum leak test (sensors removed)[a]	11.2
13.	[Sound pressure test]	10.1
	Performance qualification tests – test person	
1.	Thermometric tests for each operating cycle as required by the user	8.13

* May be done at the same time as the preceding test.

[ ] Optional test, to be done at the user's discretion.

a. For sterilizers with an active air removal system.

b. For sterilizers with an active air removal system, the PQ tests may be done at this point.

Table 3a Validation tests for high-temperature steam sterilizers

		Ref
	Commissioning tests – test person[a]	
1.	Automatic control test	12.1
2.	Verification of calibration of sterilizer instruments*	12.2
3.	Thermometric test for a full load	19.71
4.	Reheat and dispensing test	19.78

* May be done at the same time as the preceding test.

a. The commissioning tests may be omitted if test data is supplied by the manufacturer.

Table 3b Validation tests for culture media preparators

5.0 Schedule of periodic tests

Introduction

5.1 Periodic tests are carried out at daily, weekly, quarterly and yearly intervals. They are the shared responsibility of the test person and the user.

5.2 The yearly test schedule is identical to that carried out on revalidation (see paragraph 2.39). It contains tests for both recommissioning and performance requalification.

5.3 Tests should be performed on completion of planned maintenance tasks as described in Part 4. The schedules for the tests are set out for each type of clinical sterilizer in Table 4 and for laboratory sterilizers in Table 5. Each test is cross-referenced to a detailed description of the test procedure in a later chapter. The tests should be carried out with the sterilizer at normal working temperature (a warming-up cycle may be needed) and completed in the order shown.

5.4 The calibration of thermometric test equipment should be checked before and after the thermometric tests as described in Chapter 6.

5.5 Where tests on EO sterilizers require EO gas to be in the chamber, sensors should either be removed from the chamber or else disconnected from the recorder and the wires grounded to the body of the sterilizer (see note (d) to Table 4f).

5.6 The results of the tests done by the test person should be kept in the plant history file. The results of the tests done by the user should be kept in the sterilizer process log. (See Part 4 for guidance on record-keeping.)

Weekly safety checks

5.7 The test person should make the following safety checks before starting the sequence of weekly tests:

a. examine the door seal;

b. check the security and performance of door safety devices;

c. check that safety valves, or other pressure-limiting devices, are free to operate;

d. make any other checks required by the competent person in connection with the written scheme of examination for the pressure vessel.

Yearly safety checks

5.8 In order to ensure the safe functioning of the sterilizer, the test person should conduct a sequence of safety checks before starting the yearly tests. The installation checks (Chapter 3) should be used as a basis for these, but it will not be necessary to repeat them all. In selecting which checks to include in the yearly schedule, consideration should be given to conditions which affect safety and to those which may have changed over the course of time. It will not be necessary, for example, to check again that the sterilizer has been supplied in accordance with specification, but it will be necessary to check that the engineering services remain adequate and are connected safely. The authorised person should advise on which checks will need to be included.

Table 4 Schedule of periodic tests for clinical sterilizers

		Ref
	Daily test – user	
1.	Bowie-Dick test for steam penetration	13.39
	Weekly tests – test person	
1.	Weekly safety checks	5.7
2.	Vacuum leak test	11.2
3.	Air detector function test	11.60
4.	Automatic control test	12.1
5.	Bowie-Dick test for steam penetration*	13.39
	Quarterly tests – test person	
1.	Weekly safety checks	5.7
2.	Vacuum leak test	11.2
3.	Vacuum leak test (temperature and pressure sensors connected)	11.2
4.	Automatic control test	12.1
5.	Verification of calibration of sterilizer instruments*	12.2
6.	Thermometric test for a small load*	13.7
7.	Vacuum leak test (sensors removed)	11.2
8.	Air detector function test	11.60
9.	Bowie-Dick test for steam penetration	13.39
	Yearly and revalidation tests – test person	
1.	Yearly safety checks	5.8
2.	Steam non-condensable gas test	9.4
3.	Steam superheat test	9.20
4.	Steam dryness test	9.30
5.	Vacuum leak test	11.2
6.	Vacuum leak test (temperature and pressure sensors connected)	11.2
7.	Automatic control test	12.1
8.	Verification of calibration of sterilizer instruments*	12.2
9.	Air detector performance test for a small load	11.45
10.	Air detector performance test for a full load	11.53
11.	Thermometric test for a small load	13.7
12.	Tests for performance requalification as required by the user	8.64
13.	Vacuum leak test (sensors removed)	11.2
14.	Air detector function test	11.60
15.	Bowie-Dick test for steam penetration	13.39

* May be done at the same time as the preceding test.

***Table 4a* Periodic tests for porous load sterilizers**

		Ref
	Weekly tests – test person	
1.	Weekly safety checks	5.7
2.	Heat exchanger integrity test[a,b]	14.4
3.	Automatic control test	12.1
	Quarterly tests – test person	
1.	Weekly safety checks	5.7
2.	Heat exchanger integrity test[a]	14.4
3.	Automatic control test	12.1
4.	Verification of calibration of sterilizer instruments*	12.2
5.	Simplified thermometric test for performance requalification	14.27
	Yearly and revalidation tests – test person	
1.	Yearly safety checks	5.8
2.	Heat exchanger integrity test	14.4
3.	Automatic control test	12.1
4.	Verification of calibration of sterilizer instruments*	12.2
5.	Tests for performance requalification as required by the user and the quality controller (for medicinal products) or by the user (other loads)	8.64
6.	Coolant quality test	14.32

* May be done at the same time as the preceding test.

a. Not required where the heat exchanger is designed and constructed in a fail-safe fashion so that coolant in the secondary circuit cannot become contaminated in any circumstances.

b. Not required where the pressure in the secondary circuit exceeds the pressure in the primary circuit throughout the operating cycle.

Table 4b **Periodic tests for fluid sterilizers**

		Ref
	Daily test – user	
1.	Automatic control test – observe and note the reading on the cycle counter, if visible to the user	12.1
	Weekly tests – test person[a]	
1.	Weekly safety checks	5.7
2.	Automatic control test	12.1
	Quarterly tests – test person	
1.	Weekly safety checks	5.7
2.	Automatic control test	12.1
3.	Verification of calibration of sterilizer instruments*	12.2
4.	Thermometric test for a small load	15.7
	Yearly and revalidation tests – test person	
1.	Yearly safety checks	5.8
2.	Automatic control test	12.1
3.	Verification of calibration of sterilizer instruments*	12.2
4.	Chamber overheat cut-out test[b]	15.3
5.	Thermometric test for a small load	15.7
6.	Thermometric test for a full load	15.13
7.	Tests for performance requalification as required by the user	8.64

* May be done at the same time as the preceding test.

a. For transportable sterilizers, the weekly tests may be done by the user by agreement with the test person.

b. Not required where the steam is supplied from a source external to the chamber.

Table 4c **Periodic tests for sterilizers for unwrapped instruments and utensils**

		Ref
	Weekly tests – test person	
1.	Weekly safety checks	5.7
2.	Automatic control test[a]	16.4
	Quarterly tests – test person	
1.	Weekly safety checks	5.7
2.	Automatic control test	16.4
3.	Verification of calibration of sterilizer instruments*	12.2
4.	Simplified thermometric test for performance requalification	16.26
	Yearly and revalidation tests – test person	
1.	Yearly safety checks	5.8
2.	Automatic control test	16.4
3.	Verification of calibration of sterilizer instruments*	12.2
4.	Chamber overheat cut-out test	16.8
5.	Air filter integrity test	16.13
6.	Tests for performance requalification as required by the user and the quality controller (medicinal products) or by the user (other loads)	8.64

* May be done at the same time as the preceding test.

a. Not required where the previous week's batch process records are jointly reviewed by the user and the test person and, within specified limits, are comparable with previous records.

Table 4d **Periodic tests for dry-heat sterilizers**

		Ref
	Daily tests – user	
1.	Vacuum leak test[a]	11.2
2.	During the holding time of the first production cycle of the day, observe and note the reading on the cycle counter, chamber temperature indicator and chamber pressure indicator	
3.	Routine microbiological test for each production cycle (LTSF)	17.58
	Weekly tests – test person	
1.	Weekly safety checks	5.7
2.	Vacuum leak test	11.2
3.	Automatic control test	12.1
	Quarterly tests – test person	
1.	Weekly safety checks	5.7
2.	Vacuum leak test	11.2
3.	Vacuum leak test (temperature and pressure sensors connected)	11.2
4.	Automatic control test	12.1
5.	Verification of calibration of sterilizer instruments*	12.2
6.	Vacuum leak monitor test	11.19
7.	Thermometric test for a small load	17.15
8.	Vacuum leak test (sensors removed)	11.2
	Yearly and revalidation tests – test person	
1.	Yearly safety checks	5.8
2.	Vacuum leak test	11.2
3.	Vacuum leak test (temperature and pressure sensors connected)	11.2

Contd

		Ref
4.	Automatic control test	12.1
5.	Verification of calibration of sterilizer instruments*	12.2
6.	Vacuum leak monitor test	11.19
7.	Chamber overheat cut-out test	17.4
8.	Chamber wall temperature test	17.10
9.	Thermometric test for a small load	17.15
10.	Thermometric test for a full load (LTS)	17.23
11.	Microbiological test for basic performance (LTSF)	17.40
12.	Environmental formaldehyde vapour test (LTSF)	17.32
13.	Thermometric tests for performance requalification as required by the user	8.13
14.	Microbiological tests for performance requalification as required by the user (LTSF)	8.29
15.	Vacuum leak test (sensors removed)	11.2
	Yearly and revalidation tests – user	
1.	Tests for degassing time (LTSF, performance requalification)	8.46

* May be done at the same time as the preceding test.
a. Not required where a vacuum leak monitor is fitted.

Table 4e **Periodic tests for LTS disinfectors and LTSF sterilizers**

		Ref
	Daily tests – user	
1.	Routine microbiological test for each production cycle	18.58
	Weekly tests – test person	
1.	Weekly safety checks	5.7
2.	Vacuum leak test	11.2
3.	Pressure leak test[a]	11.24
4.	Automatic control test[b]	12.1
	Quarterly tests – test person	
1.	Weekly safety checks	5.7
2.	Vacuum leak test	11.2
3.	Pressure leak test[a]	11.24
4.	Vacuum leak test (temperature and pressure sensors connected)	11.2
5.	Pressure leak test[a]	11.24
6.	Automatic control test	12.1
7.	Verification of calibration of sterilizer instruments*	12.2
8.	Vacuum leak monitor test	11.19
9.	Chamber space temperature test	18.11
10.	Vacuum leak test (sensors removed)	11.2
11.	Pressure leak test[a]	11.24
	Yearly and revalidation tests – test person	
1.	Yearly safety checks	5.8
2.	Vacuum leak test	11.2
3.	Pressure leak test[a]	11.24
4.	Vacuum leak test (temperature, pressure and humidity sensors connected)	11.2

Contd

		Ref
5.	Pressure leak test[a]	11.24
6.	Automatic control test	12.1
7.	Verification of calibration of sterilizer instruments*	12.2
8.	Vacuum leak monitor test	11.19
9.	Chamber overheat cut-out test	18.4
10.	Chamber wall temperature test	18.16
11.	Chamber space temperature test	18.11
12.	Gas circulation test[c,d]	
13.	Microbiological test for basic performance[d]	18.30
14.	Thermometric tests for performance requalification as required by the user	18.36
15.	Microbiological tests for performance requalification as required by the user[b]	18.49
16.	Environmental gas tests*,[d]	8.37
17.	Vacuum leak test (sensors removed)	11.2
18.	Pressure leak test[a]	11.24
	Yearly and revalidation tests – user	
1.	Tests for degassing time (performance requalification)	8.46

* May be done at the same time as the preceding test.

a. Required only where the sterilizer operates above atmospheric pressure.

b. Not required where the previous week's batch process records are jointly reviewed by the user and the test person and, within specified limits, are comparable with previous records.

c. Required only where a circulating fan is fitted. Instrumentation is used to demonstrate that pressures and flows specified by the manufacturer are obtained.

d. To avoid risk of sparking, tests using EO gas should not be done while temperature sensors are in the chamber. Providing safe operating procedures are not compromised, it may be acceptable to disconnect the sensors from the recorder and ground the wires to the body of the sterilizer.

Table 4f **Periodic tests for ethylene oxide sterilizers**

Table 5 Schedule of periodic tests for laboratory sterilizers

		Ref
	Daily tests – user	
1.	During the holding time of the first production cycle of the day, observe and note the reading on the cycle counter, chamber temperature indicator and chamber pressure indicator	
	Weekly tests – test person	
1.	Weekly safety checks	5.7
2.	Vacuum leak test[a]	11.2
3.	Automatic control test[b]	12.1
	Quarterly tests – test person	
1.	Weekly safety checks	5.7
2.	Vacuum leak test[a]	11.2
3.	Vacuum leak test (temperature and pressure sensors connected)[a]	11.2
4.	Automatic control test for each operating cycle	12.1
5.	Verification of calibration of sterilizer instruments*	12.2

Contd

		Ref
6.	Thermometric test for a small load (small plastic discard, or fabrics, or glassware and equipment)[c]	19.16, 13.7, 19.61
7.	Simplified thermometric test for performance requalification (contained fluid discard, or culture media, or free steaming)[c]	19.46
8.	Vacuum leak test (sensors removed)[a]	11.2
9.	Thermal door-lock override test	19.64
	Yearly and revalidation tests – test person	
1.	Yearly safety checks	5.8
2.	Vacuum leak test[a]	11.2
3.	Vacuum leak test (temperature and pressure sensors connected)[a]	11.2
4.	Automatic control test for each operating cycle	12.1
5.	Verification of calibration of sterilizer instruments*	12.2
6.	Thermometric test for a small load (small plastic discard, or fabrics, or glassware and equipment)[c]	19.16, 13.7, 19.61
7.	Thermometric test for a full load (contained fluid discard, or culture media, or free steaming)[c]	19.24
8.	Tests for performance requalification as required by the user	8.64
9.	Vacuum leak test (sensors removed)[a]	11.2
10.	Thermal door-lock override test	19.64

* May be done at the same time as the preceding test.
a. Required only for sterilizers with an active air removal system.
b. The cycle should be chosen on a rotating basis from the cycles in routine use.
c. Required only for the first cycle listed in brackets that is available on the sterilizer.

Table 5a **Periodic tests for high-temperature steam sterilizers**

		Ref
	Weekly tests – user or test person	
1.	Weekly safety checks	5.7
2.	Automatic control test	12.1
	Yearly tests – test person	
1.	Yearly safety checks	5.8
2.	Automatic control test	12.1
3.	Verification of calibration of sterilizer instruments*	12.2
4.	Thermometric test for a full load	19.71
5.	Reheat and dispensing test	19.78

* May be done at the same time as the preceding test.

Table 5b **Periodic tests for culture media preparators**

6.0 Test equipment

Introduction

6.1 This chapter discusses the portable test equipment required to carry out the test procedures described in this document. Specifications for instruments fitted permanently to sterilizers are given in the relevant British and European Standards discussed in Part 2 of this HTM.

6.2 With the rapid advance in instrumentation technology, it is becoming increasingly difficult (and undesirable) to set detailed specifications for the equipment to be used in testing sterilizers. For example, a clear trend is for much of the testing to be under the control of a computer which can automatically take the desired measurements, check that they meet the requirements of the tests in this HTM, and report the results. The object of this chapter is twofold. First, to ensure that the traditional measurement methods are adequately supported; and second, to make clear the essential requirements for test equipment that apply for old and new technology alike. Where it is proposed to use measurement and recording techniques that are not explicitly covered here, the advice of the authorised person should be sought.

6.3 Access to standard laboratory equipment and supplies is assumed.

Calibration and sources of error

6.4 The errors produced in temperature and pressure measurement will arise from a number of factors. Some are inherent in the design, age and condition of the measuring equipment, and others are due to loose terminals, imperfect plug and socket connections, and the change of environmental temperature around the instrument. Variations in thermocouple alloys, preparation of thermocouple hot junctions, the method of introducing sensors into the chamber, and their location within the load will add to the error in temperature measurement. Temperature fluctuations within pressure-sensing elements will lead to errors in pressure measurement.

6.5 Every effort should be made to eliminate or minimise these errors by attention to detail, location of instruments, effective maintenance, and skill in the application, handling and use of the instruments. Systematic errors can be reduced by careful calibration.

6.6 Instruments should be maintained and calibrated as recommended by the manufacturer as part of a planned maintenance programme. Each instrument should be labelled with the calibration date and a reference to its certificate. The calibration of all test instruments should be verified yearly by using reference instruments with a valid certificate of calibration traceable to a national standard. A history record should be kept for each instrument.

6.7 All electronic test instruments should be allowed a period of time to stabilize within the test site environment. They should be located in a position protected from draughts, and should not be subjected to rapid temperature variations. The manufacturer's instructions should be followed.

Recorders

6.8 Test recorders are required to measure temperature and pressure in all types of sterilizer, and humidity in EO sterilizers. They should be designed for use with the appropriate sensors, independent of those fitted to the sterilizer, as described later in this chapter. Most of the tests in this HTM may be conducted with a single recorder combining temperature and pressure functions, preferably showing both records on the same chart or print-out. For EO sterilizers, a third function, for humidity, is desirable but not essential.

6.9 Twelve temperature channels are sufficient for all the tests on each type of sterilizer in this HTM, though more may be convenient for determining chamber temperature profiles (see paragraph 7.21). One pressure channel is required for all sterilizers except fluid sterilizers which require up to three. The pressure channel for a dry-heat sterilizer is required to measure the small differential pressure (no more than 10 mbar) across the air filter. Two relative-humidity channels are desirable for EO sterilizers.

6.10 Analogue recorders (conventional pen and chart recorders) should comply with the display requirements of BS3693. If they use potentiometric techniques, they should comply with BS5164.

6.11 Digital recorders (data loggers) are rapidly coming into use and have many advantages over traditional pen recorders. They measure the variables electronically and store the values in digital form suitable for computer processing. Data may be presented graphically or as a numerical list, or as a combination of both. Parts of the operating cycle, such as the plateau period, can be expanded and replotted for closer examination. The record should quantify all turning points in the data, and distinguish by colour, print format or separate list, measurements which are within the sterilization temperature band for the operating cycle under test. The recorder should have the facility for downloading data onto tape or disk which can then be removed and kept securely. Software used with digital recorders should be developed under a quality system (such as BS5750) and validated before use.

6.12 The detailed specification for a test recorder will depend upon the range of sterilizers with which it is to be used. In all cases the recorder and its sensors should be capable of measuring cycle variables to considerably greater accuracy than the instruments fitted to the sterilizer.

6.13 The accuracy with which a variable can be read from the recorder will be affected not only by the sources of error discussed above (see paragraph 6.4), but also by the precision of the calibration, the scale range selected, the integration time, the sampling interval and the intrinsic accuracy of the recorder itself. Digital recorders will invariably register measurements to a precision greater than the accuracy of the system as a whole, and care should be taken in interpreting such measurements.

6.14 The intrinsic accuracies quoted by recorder manufacturers are measured under controlled reference conditions and do not include errors from temperature, pressure or humidity sensors. Temperature measurement errors due to ambient temperature changes should not exceed 0.04°C per °C rise.

6.15 The scale ranges should include the expected maximum and minimum values of the cycle variables throughout the operating cycle, with sufficient leeway to accommodate any deviations resulting from a malfunctioning sterilizer. (Note that in some sterilizers the temperature in the chamber free space will considerably exceed the upper limit of the sterilization temperature band for a short time at the start of the plateau period.)

6.16 The most critical stage of the operating cycle is the plateau period (the equilibration time plus the holding time, see paragraph 7.11) during which the load becomes exposed to the sterilization conditions. It is during this period that the values of the cycle variables are at their most critical and the recorder should be capable of measuring them to sufficient accuracy to confirm that the sterilization conditions have been attained. The criteria are as follows:

a. for digital recorders, the sampling interval should be short enough for the holding time to contain at least 180 independent measurements in each recording channel. This corresponds to a sampling interval of one second for the shortest holding time (3 minute, high-temperature steam sterilizers) and 40 seconds for the longest (120 minute, dry-heat sterilizers). For pen recorders, the chart speed should be fast enough to allow fluctuations on that scale to be clearly resolved. The duration of the holding time should be measurable to within 1%;

b. the integration time of the recorder (the response time) should be short enough to enable the output to follow significant fluctuations in the cycle variables and to ensure that successive measurements are independent of each other. It should not be longer than the sampling interval;

c. the width of the sterilization temperature band (see paragraph 7.14) varies from 3°C (high-temperature steam sterilizers) to 10°C (dry-heat sterilizers). The recorder must be accurate enough to show clearly whether the measured temperatures are within the band or not. For all the types of sterilizer covered by this HTM, the repeatability of the recorder should be ± 0.25°C or better, and the limit of error of the complete measurement system (including sensors) should be no more than 0.5°C;

d. for pressure measurement, the limit of error should be no more than 0.5% of the absolute pressure during the plateau period;

e. for humidity measurement, the limiting factor is likely to be the performance of the sensor (see paragraph 6.47).

6.17 A recorder chosen to meet these criteria for the plateau period will have more than enough performance for the preceding and following stages of the operating cycle.

6.18 If a fluid sterilizer is fitted with an F_0 integrating system (see Part 4 for a discussion of the use of F_0 in controlling operating cycles), then the recorder should be capable of computing and printing values of F_0 for each channel with integration times no greater than 2 s (see BS3970: Part 2).

Temperature measurement

Temperature sensors

6.19 Temperature sensors are required to sense the temperature in locations in the chamber and load as specified in the tests. They may be either platinum resistance elements or thermocouples.

6.20 Platinum resistance elements should comply with Class A of BS1904.

6.21 Thermocouples should conform to BS4937: Part 4 (nickel-chromium/nickel-aluminium) or Part 5 (copper/constantan). The calibration accuracy should be Tolerance Class 1 as specified in EN 60584: Part 2 (formerly BS4937: Part 20). The tolerance on Part 4 thermocouples (± 1.5°C) is high when compared with that allowed for those in Part 5 (± 0.5°C), and for this reason copper/constantan thermocouples are usually preferred for the test recording system.

6.22 Thermocouple wire is available which is marked to show the limits of variation of the reel from the figures given in the British Standard. The variation will have been established by the manufacturer by testing samples from both ends of the full reel. "Selected" rather than "standard" wire should be used. For "selected" wire this variation is typically (for copper/constantan) of the order of 0.015 mV which is equivalent to 0.4°C at 20°C and 0.3°C at 134°C.

6.23 The wire should be single-strand, not exceeding 0.7 mm diameter over the covering of one core of a twin cable. Twin-core cable is usually preferred because it is easier to handle and more durable than single-core wire. The width of the cable should not exceed 2 mm. If bulkier cable is used, the tracking of steam along the outside of the cable may invalidate certain tests, such as those which require temperatures to be measured in the centre of a standard test pack (see paragraph 7.27).

6.24 Thermocouples may be argon arc-welded or micro-welded. However, experience has shown that provided the wires are cleaned, they may be satisfactorily twisted together to form the hot junction. Brazing, silver brazing and welding with filler rods may be no more reliable in respect of accuracy than freshly twisted wires. Particular attention should be given to the condition of copper/constantan thermocouples when testing LTSF sterilizers. Thermocouples should not be fitted with a heat sink.

Use of sensors

6.25 A typical method of introducing sensors into a sterilizer chamber is illustrated in Figure 2. Methods which prevent the removal of individual sensors are to be discouraged. In older machines having no dedicated entry port, entry may be made via a tee which can usually be inserted into a service entry pipe to the chamber (for example the steam supply pipe). Sensors should not be introduced through the door seal. The test schedules for sterilizers employing active air removal systems provide for a vacuum leak test to be done after temperature sensors have been introduced into the chamber, and again after they have been removed, to ensure that the chamber remains gas-tight.

6.26 Many of the tests require a temperature sensor to be placed in the active chamber discharge of the sterilizer. This is a drain or vent which permits the controlled flow of air and condensate (a drain) or of air alone (a vent), such that the temperature within the discharge is the same as the chamber temperature. The preferred locations are as follows:

a. in the drain, if it is active throughout the operating cycle;

b. otherwise in a vent, if it is active throughout the operating cycle;

c. otherwise in the coldest part of the usable chamber space.

6.27 The sensor should be placed in the drain or vent in steam phase boundary conditions in a position where overheat cannot be detected. This will normally require at least 10 mm insertion depth. The sensors connected to the sterilizer temperature indicator and recorder, and to the automatic controller, are normally in this position also. Care should be taken to ensure that the sensor does not touch any metal parts. (Contact between the hot junction and metal surfaces can cause induced electromotive forces (EMFs) leading to inaccurate readings.)

6.28 Figure 3 shows several methods for inserting sensors into glass or plastic containers filled with fluid or powders. It is important that the sensor is firmly supported and that the container does not leak. For rigid containers the sensor should be located on the vertical axis and inserted to a depth of 85 ± 5% of the height of the container. For flexible containers, such as plastic bags, the sensor should be located as near as practicable to the centre of the fluid and supported in this position throughout the operating cycle.

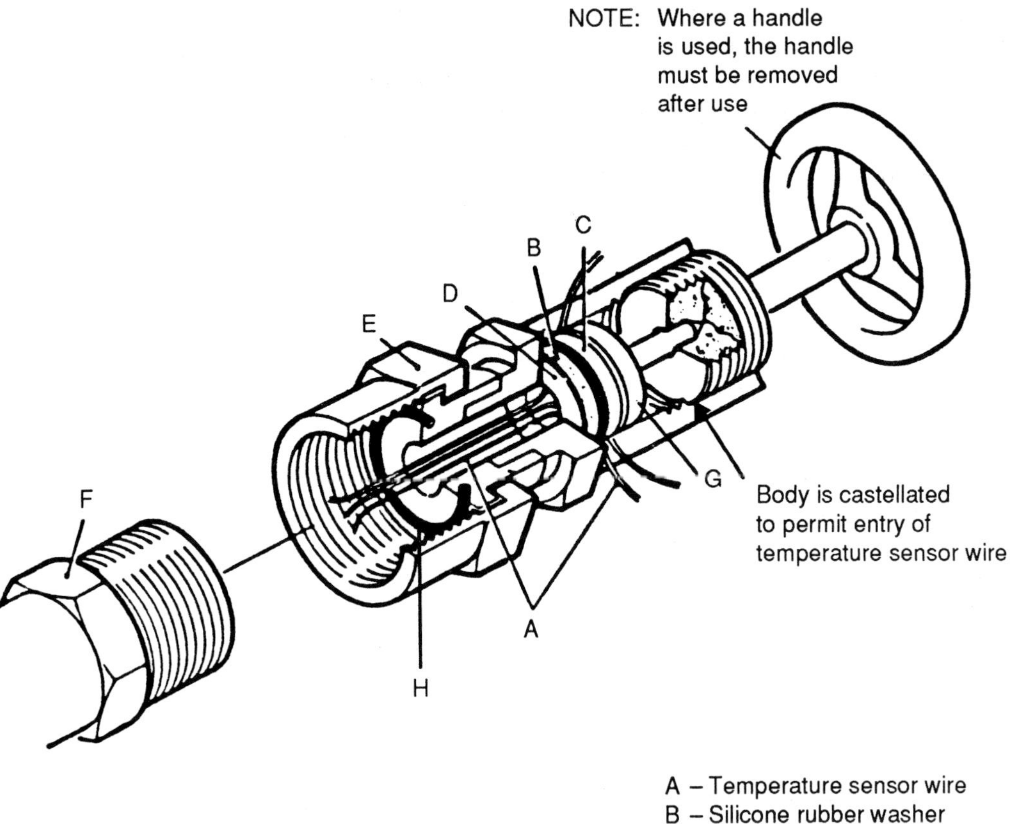

A – Temperature sensor wire
B – Silicone rubber washer
C – Silicone rubber disc
D – Metal thrust washer
E – Metal body
F – Adaptor
G – Metal thrust spigot
H – O-ring

The illustration shows a fitting designed for a sterilizing chamber having a male gland and an 'O' ring seal. When the gland is a female thread an adaptor will be required (F). Other methods of introducing temperature sensors into a sterilizer chamber and which guarantee a gas-tight seal are equally acceptable.

Figure 2 A method of introducing temperature sensors into a sterilizer chamber

6.29 When sensors are used in fluid containers, steam or fluid may be forced along the wire between the core and the sheath. To prevent damage to the recorder, the outer sheath should be either punctured a few centimetres from the end or stripped back for a similar distance to ensure that droplets forming where the sheath has been punctured or terminated fall clear of the recorder.

6.30 If the load item is a solid object, the sensor should be held securely in good thermal contact with the object.

6.31 Where required, sensors may be attached to the chamber walls by means of masking tape.

Container entry system

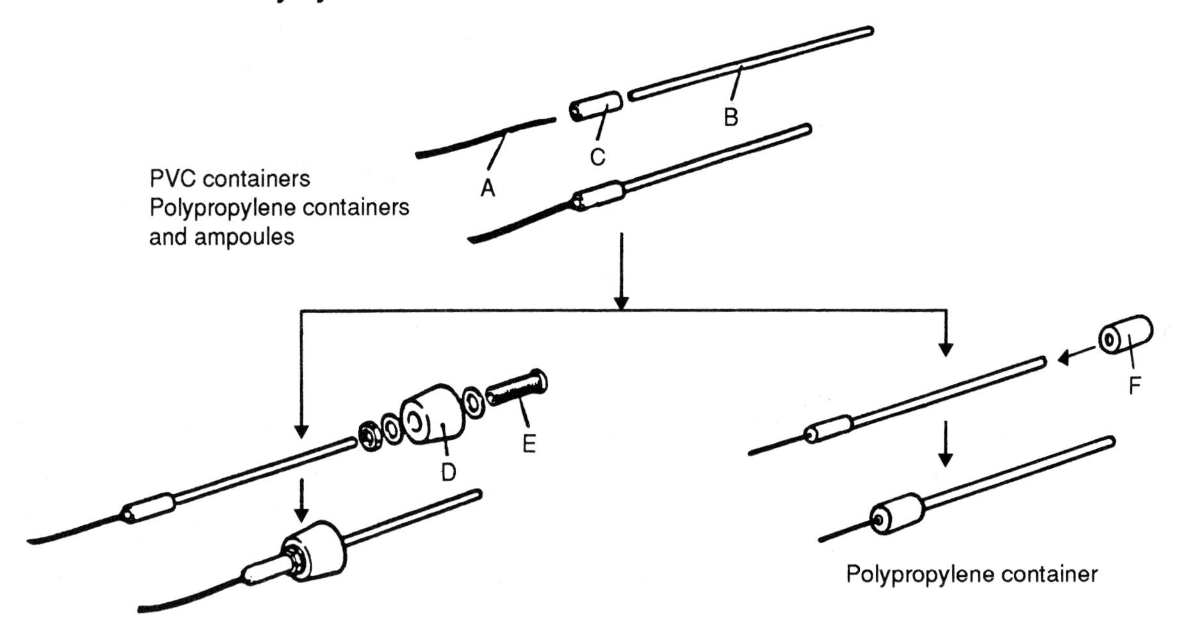

DIN containers and others

A – Temperature sensor, wire 2mm O/D
B – Needle tubing, 12 SWG, sealed at one end only
C – Silicone tubing, 4,5mm O/D x 1mm I/D
D – No. 21 rubber stopper (BS2775) with 8mm diameter bore (used for DIN containers)
E – Gland assembly (M8 x 25mm bolt with 5mm bore)
F – Silicone tubing (to suit container)

Examples

A – DIN standard glass
B – Glass ampoules
C – Rigid plastic container
D – Flexible plastic container

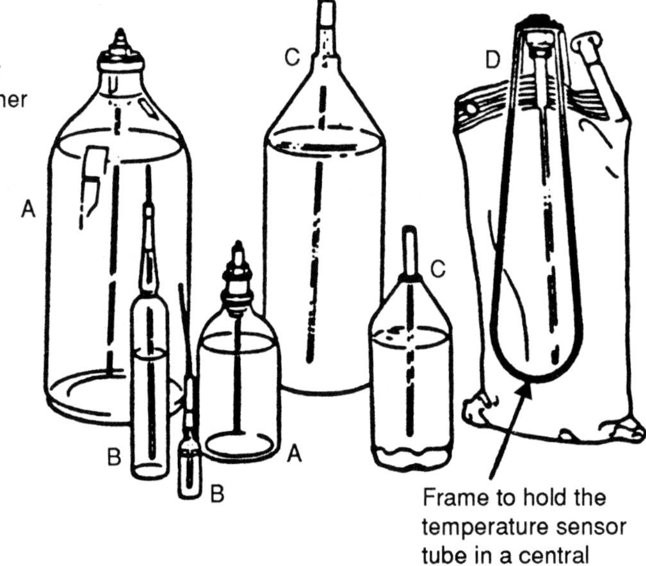

Figure 3 Methods of inserting temperature sensors into load containers

Verification of calibration

6.32 The recorder should incorporate mechanical or electrical calibration facilities. The manufacturer of the recorder will normally calibrate it without the use of temperature sensors or transducers.

6.33 An independent temperature reference source (a "hot source") is required, with a pocket to accommodate up to 12 temperature sensors. The temperature gradient within the pocket should not exceed 0.2°C and the control accuracy should be within ± 0.1°C over the relevant sterilization temperature band.

6.34 The temperature of the hot source should be measured either by a mercury-in-glass laboratory thermometer conforming to BS593 or other temperature measurement system of similar or greater accuracy. The supplier should be asked to provide a certified calibration curve traceable to the national primary standard. Note that all the thermometric measurements required by this HTM will ultimately depend upon the accuracy of this calibration; an uncertified laboratory thermometer will not be accurate enough to ensure that the sterilizer is working correctly and may give dangerously misleading results. The following types of mercury-in-glass thermometers are suitable:

a. F 75C/100 (24°C to 78°C) for EO sterilizers;

b. F 100C/100 (48°C to 102°C) for LTS disinfectors and LTSF sterilizers;

c. F 150C/100 (98°C to 152°C) for high-temperature steam sterilizers;

d. F 200C/100 (148°C to 202°C) for dry-heat sterilizers.

6.35 Mercury-in-glass thermometers should be used only in the hot source and must never be placed inside a sterilizer chamber. Note that mercury-in-glass thermometers are not permitted to be taken into pharmaceutical production facilities.

6.36 Before a recorder is taken to site, verify the calibration of the system by inserting the test sensors into the hot source at a temperature within the sterilization temperature band. Adjust the recorder in accordance with the manufacturer's instructions until the mean temperature measured by the sensors is the same as the temperature indicated on the thermometer. The calibration is satisfactory if the temperatures measured by individual sensors do not differ from the mean by more than 0.5°C. This test should be carried out at an ambient temperature as close as practicable to that expected at site.

6.37 If the hot source is not to be taken to site, connect a millivolt source to one channel of the recorder, and adjust it until the measured temperature is within 2°C of that obtained with the sensors connected. Note the measured temperature and the voltage indicated on the millivolt source. Also note the ambient air temperature near the source.

6.38 After arriving at site, and before starting any thermometric tests, check the calibration using either the hot source or the millivolt source.

a. If the hot source is used, adjust the temperature to correspond with that used off-site. Check that each sensor is measuring the same temperature as before;

b. If the millivolt source is used, ensure that the ambient temperature is similar to that measured off-site. Connect the millivolt source to the recorder, apply the voltage obtained off-site and check that the same temperature is measured. Bundle all the sensors together, place them in the chamber and expose them to an operating cycle. Check that the temperatures measured during the holding time are consistent with those obtained off-site with the hot source.

6.39 Repeat the check after the tests have been completed.

Pressure measurement

6.40 Pressures are required to be measured over a range from 20 mbar absolute (in vacuum leak testing) to typically 3.8 bar absolute at the working pressure of a high-temperature steam sterilizer and 7 bar absolute at the working pressure of a sterilizer using EO gas diluted with carbon dioxide.

Transducers

6.41 Transducers for use with pressure recorders should conform with BS6447, be suitable for the purpose, certified and no less accurate than the gauges specified below. The natural frequency of the sensor and connected tubing should not be less than 10 Hz, and the time constant for rising pressure (0–63%) should not be greater than 0.04 s.

Gauges

6.42 Pressure gauges are required where the pressure recorder is unsuitable or for calibrating pressure instruments fitted to the sterilizer. Four gauges will normally be required to cover the whole pressure range for all sterilizers and these are specified in Table 6.

Scale range [bar]	Mark interval [mbar]	Calibration	Application
0 to 0.160 (abs)	1	Gas	Vacuum leak testing
–1 to 0	10	Gas	LTS, LTSF + pure EO cycles
0 to 4	50	Liquid	High-temp steam, EO + HFC cycles
0 to 10	200	Gas	EO + CO_2 cycles

Table 6 Pressure gauges for test purposes

6.43 Pressure gauges should be temperature-compensated and, except for the absolute gauge, be Bourdon-tube test gauges conforming to EN 837: Part 1 of nominal size 150 mm and accuracy class 0.25 (that is, the error should not exceed 0.25% of the maximum scale range). For pressure leak testing on EO sterilizers, gauges should be of accuracy class 1 or, better, over a range within 10% of the gas exposure pressure.

6.44 Gauges not designed for direct connection to steam at 2.8 bar should be connected via a syphon or similar device to ensure that the accuracy of the gauge is maintained over the temperature range associated with changing steam pressure. If the low-pressure gauge used for vacuum leak testing cannot withstand the pressure in the chamber during sterilization an automatic valve should be provided to protect it.

6.45 Gauges should be tested yearly by a recognised testing laboratory as described in paragraph 5.2.1 of BS1780.

6.46 The very low differential pressure across the air filter in a dry-heat sterilizer can be measured with a water manometer with a range of up to 10 mbar.

Humidity measurement

6.47 Humidity is a critical cycle variable in the control of EO processes. The level of humidity in the chamber and load at the end of the conditioning stage is ideally measured during validation by test instruments calibrated for relative humidity (RH) at atmospheric pressure. The accuracy of measurement should not be less than ± 10% RH over the range 30–80% RH.

6.48 In practice, the measurement of relative humidity within the chamber of an EO sterilizer is difficult. Although the new European Standard on EO sterilizers will require RH sensors to be fitted, such sensors are still rare in the UK and the NHS has little experience in their use. If suitable test sensors are not available, then the chamber humidity may be validated by calculation as discussed in Appendix 2.

6.49 There is no British Standard for humidity sensors, but it is recommended that test sensors should function at temperatures of 10–60°C and at pressures from vacuum up to 7 bar absolute.

6.50 The sensitivity and accuracy of electrically operated humidity sensors is often compromised by exposure to EO. The tests described in this HTM require humidity to be measured only during cycles where an inert substitute for EO is used. The measurement can then be extrapolated to production cycles provided the other cycle variables are the same. If it becomes necessary to measure the humidity during cycles using EO gas, sensors should normally be replaced, degassed and recalibrated after each cycle.

Other instruments

Sound level meter

6.51 An integrating-averaging sound level meter is required for the sound pressure test. It should comply with Type 2 of BS6698. Ten microphones are required for a single sterilizer.

Air flow metering device

6.52 A metering device (such as a needle valve) is required to admit air into the sterilizer chamber for the air detector tests, and vacuum and pressure leak tests. The device should be capable of controlling the flow of air into an evacuated chamber. It should be adjustable and have a range which includes a flow of 0–5 ml min^{-1} per litre volume of the sterilizer chamber. The error in repeatability between 10% and 90% of the setting range should not exceed ± 5%. The device is connected to the chamber by a valved port provided by the sterilizer manufacturer.

Balance

6.53 A laboratory balance is required for steam dryness tests, load dryness tests and coolant quality tests. It should be capable of measuring the mass of loads up to 2 kg to an accuracy of 0.1 g (dryness tests), and up to 100 g to an accuracy of 0.1 mg (coolant quality test).

Gas monitoring instrument

6.54 A gas monitoring instrument, such as an infrared spectrophotometer, is required for tests on LTSF and EO sterilizers.

6.55 The formaldehyde instrument should be suitable for measuring formaldehyde concentration in air with an accuracy of ± 10% at 2 ppm.

6.56 The ethylene oxide instrument should be suitable for measuring ethylene oxide concentration in air with an accuracy of ± 10% at 15 ppm.

6.57 The scale ranges should include the appropriate short-term exposure limits specified in Table 1, and extend to at least ten times the exposure limit. The two functions may be combined in one instrument.

Aerosol generator

6.58 An aerosol generator is required for tests on dry-heat sterilizers.

6.59 The device should be capable of generating a polydisperse aerosol with particles having the size distribution shown in Table 7.

Particle size [μm]	Fraction by mass [%]
< 0.5	> 20
< 0.7	> 50
< 1.0	> 75

Source: BS5295: Part 1

Table 7 Particle size distribution for aerosol generator

Photometer

6.60 A photometer is required for tests on dry-heat sterilizers.

6.61 The device should be suitable for estimation or comparison of mass concentration of airborne particles as defined in Table 7. It should have an accuracy of better than ± 5% over the range of a five-expandable, six-decade resolution (that is, 0.01% to 100% of the test cloud) as specified in Appendix C of BS5295: Part 1.

6.62 The photometer should have a minimum threshold sensitivity of 0.0001 $\mu g\ l^{-1}$ and should be capable of measuring aerosol concentration in the range 80–120 $\mu g\ l^{-1}$.

6.63 The sample flow rate should be 0.40 ± 0.05 $l\ s^{-1}$ and sampling should be via a suitable probe device.

7.0 Testing methods

Introduction

7.1 This chapter discusses general principles and methods that are used in the thermometric and microbiological tests described in this HTM.

Terminology

7.2 For the purposes of this HTM the following definitions have been adopted.

Cycle variables

7.3 The **cycle variables** are the physical properties, such as time, temperature, pressure, humidity and sterilant gas concentration, that influence the efficacy of the sterilization process. Most of the tests described in this HTM require the values of cycle variables to be determined experimentally and then compared with standard values.

7.4 An **indicated** value is that shown by a dial or other visual display fitted permanently to the sterilizer.

7.5 A **recorded** value is that shown on the output of a recording instrument fitted permanently to the sterilizer.

7.6 A **measured** value is that shown on a test instrument, such as a thermometric recorder or a test pressure gauge, attached to the sterilizer for test purposes.

7.7 A **noted** value is that written down by the operator, usually as the result of observing an indicated, recorded or measured value.

Sterilization conditions

7.8 Most operating cycles have a stage in which the load is exposed to the sterilization (or disinfection) conditions for a specified length of time. This period is known as the **holding time**.

7.9 The **sterilization conditions** are the ranges of the cycle variables which may prevail throughout the chamber and load during the holding time.

7.10 The holding time is preceded by a period in which the sterilization conditions are present in the chamber but not yet present throughout the load. This is known as the **equilibration time**.

7.11 Together, the equilibration time and the holding time constitute the **plateau period**. While the plateau period can always be determined from the recorded chamber temperature, the equilibration and holding times cannot be distinguished unless the temperature in the part of the load that is slowest to reach the sterilization temperature is also being recorded or measured.

7.12 Certain LTSF sterilizers may achieve sterilization by exposing the load to a series of pulses of formaldehyde rather than a single holding time.

7.13 For EO sterilizers the plateau period is equivalent to the **gas exposure time.** The holding time cannot be determined by thermometry and is therefore of no practical interest.

7.14 For steam and dry-heat sterilizers, the sterilization conditions are specified by a **sterilization temperature band**, defined by a minimum acceptable temperature, known as the **sterilization temperature**, and a maximum allowable temperature. A sterilization temperature band can also be quoted for LTSF and EO sterilizers, but since these processes depend primarily upon chemical action such a band is not a complete specification of the sterilization conditions. Bands for the different types of sterilizer are listed in Table 8.

	High-temperature steam				Dry heat			LTS	LTSF	Ethylene oxide
Sterilization temperature [°C][a]	115	121	126	134	160	170	180	71[b]	71	30–56
Maximum allowable temperature [°C]	118	124	129	137	170	180	190	80	80	T^{c}
Minimum holding time [min]	30	15	10	3	120	60	30	10	180[d]	t^{e}

a. The temperature setting on the automatic controller will not generally be the sterilization temperature, but a higher temperature within the sterilization temperature band.
b. Disinfection temperature.
c. For EO, the maximum allowable temperature will normally be 4°C above the sterilization temperature.
d. For LTSF, the sterilization conditions may specify either a continuous holding time or the number of pulses of formaldehyde required to achieve sterilization.
e. For EO, the "gas exposure time" is determined for each sterilizer by microbiological methods during commissioning but is typically 2–7 h depending upon sterilization temperature and gas concentration.

Table 8 Sterilization temperature bands

Interpretation of thermometric measurements

7.15 Figure 4 shows in schematic form the kind of data that are typically obtained in a thermometric test using measuring equipment as described in Chapter 6. In practice there may be more or fewer temperature traces depending on the number of sensors used. The detailed behaviour before and after the plateau period is dependent on the nature of the operating cycle and is not shown here.

7.16 The equilibration time begins when the temperature in the coolest part of the chamber (normally the active chamber discharge, see paragraph 6.26) first attains the sterilization temperature. It ends when the holding time begins.

7.17 The holding time begins when the temperature in the part of the load that is the slowest to heat up first attains the sterilization temperature. It ends at the start of the cooling stage, when the temperature in the coolest part of the chamber falls below the sterilization temperature.

7.18 The **fluctuation** in a trace over a given interval is $\pm T$ °C if the difference between the maximum and minimum values is $2T$.

7.19 The **drift** in a trace over a given interval is the change in the mean value of the trace over that interval.

7.20 The **difference** between two traces is the difference in their values at a given instant. A trace is said to be **within** T °C of a given value or another trace if the difference between them at any instant over a given interval is no more than T.

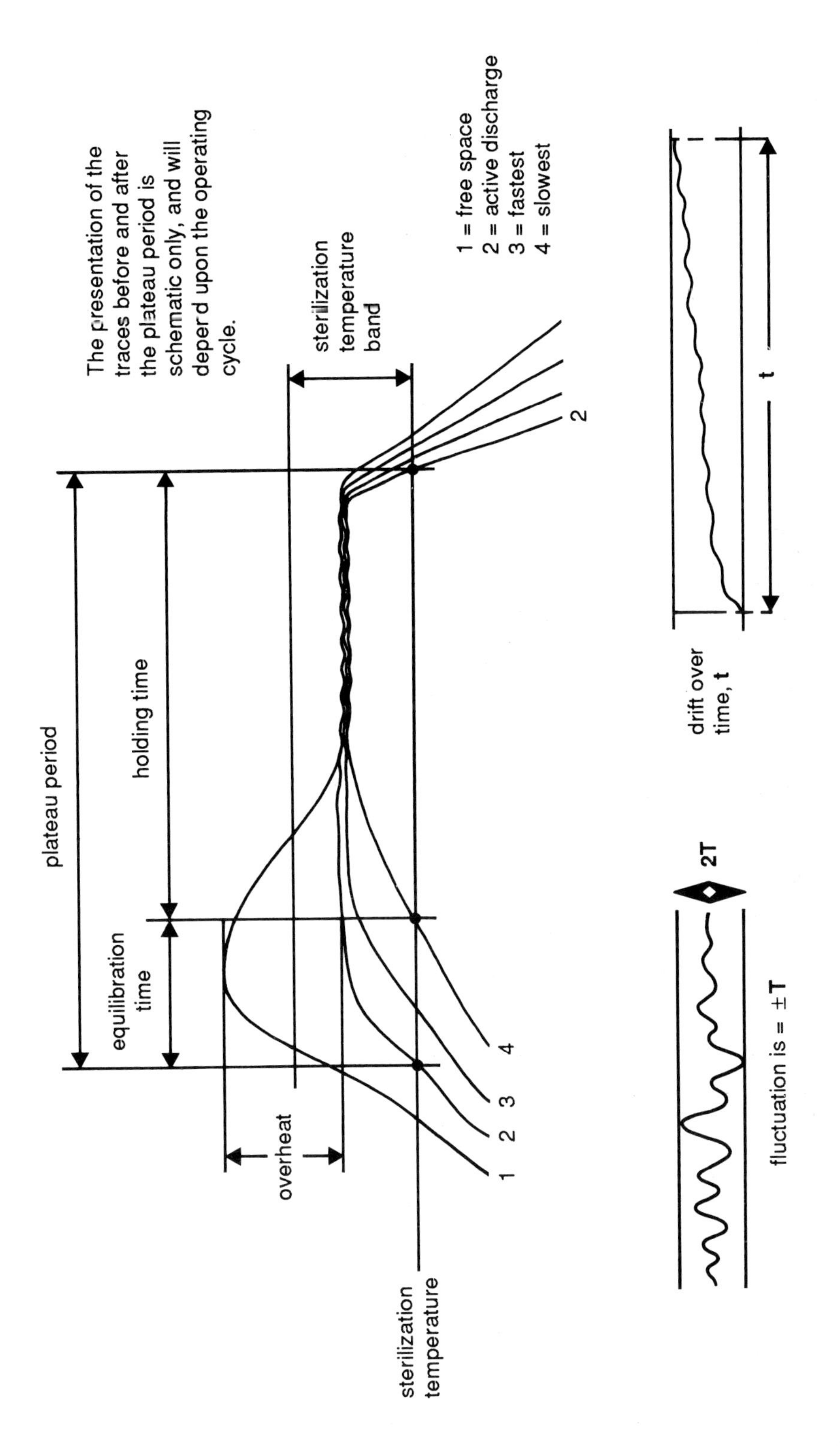

Figure 4 Interpretation of thermometric recording

Chamber temperature profile

7.21 Many of the tests require temperature sensors (or biological or chemical indicators) to be placed in the parts of the load known to be the most difficult to sterilize. To make this assessment, it is necessary to know the hottest and coolest parts of the chamber, and the parts that are the fastest and slowest to attain the sterilization temperature.

7.22 This procedure is not required for porous load sterilizers since compliance with the small-load, full-load and air detector tests ensures that the penetration of steam is effectively instantaneous.

7.23 Place temperature sensors on a grid pattern throughout the usable chamber space. The number of sensors should be at least as many as that specified for the relevant full-load test. If the test recorder has too few channels it will be necessary to run through more than one operating cycle to collect data from a sufficient number of points. If so, at least two sensors should remain in the same positions (including one in an active chamber discharge) to establish the correlation between successive cycles.

7.24 If a choice of operating cycles is available, select the cycle with the highest sterilization temperature. This will normally be 134°C for high-temperature steam sterilizers. Start the cycle.

7.25 At the end of the cycle, examine the measured temperatures and note the following:

a. the parts of the usable chamber space that are the fastest and the slowest to attain the sterilization temperature;

b. the parts of the usable chamber space that are the hottest and the coolest during the sterilization holding time;

c. for sterilizers with a thermal door interlock, the part of the usable chamber space that is the slowest to cool to 80°C.

7.26 users should be aware that the temperature profile derived in this way is valid only for an empty chamber. The presence of a load will disturb the profile, although the positions determined in paragraph 7.25 will be accurate enough for most practical purposes. However, where the sterilizer is to be used to process medicinal products, the positions will need to be confirmed for each loading condition as part of the performance qualification procedure (see paragraph 8.17).

Standard test pack

7.27 In order to ensure that tests are carried out under repeatable conditions, European Standards require the use of a "standard test pack" for all sterilizers designed to process porous loads. As well as porous load sterilizers themselves, the standard test pack is used for tests on LTS disinfectors, LTSF sterilizers and laboratory sterilizers with a cycle for the disinfection of fabrics.

7.28 The standard test pack is used to check that, at the levels at which the cycle variables are set, rapid and even penetration of steam into the pack is attained. The pack is chosen to represent the maximum density of porous load material which a sterilizer conforming to British and European Standards should be able to process. It may be used with other materials to form a full load.

7.29 The test pack is composed of plain cotton sheets complying with BS5815: Part 1, each bleached to a good white and having an approximate size of 90 cm

× 120 cm. The number of threads per centimetre in the warp should be 30 ± 6 and in the weft 27 ± 5.

7.30 The sheets should be washed but not subjected to any conditioning agent. (Conditioning agents may affect the characteristics of the fabric and may contain volatile substances which will contribute to the non-condensable gases in the chamber.)

7.31 The sheets should be dried and then aired for at least one hour at a temperature of 15–25°C and a relative humidity of 30–70%. Failure to observe this protocol can result in the test giving a pass result when it should have been a failure. Sheets which have become excessively dehydrated may cause superheating in the pack, which might also produce misleading results.

7.32 After airing, the sheets should be folded to approximately 22 cm × 30 cm and stacked to a height of approximately 25 cm. After being compressed by hand, the pack should be wrapped in similar fabric and then secured with tape no more than 25 mm wide. The total weight of the pack should be 7.0 ± 0.7 kg. The sheets will become compressed after the pack has been used. If the weight of sheets needed to form a stack 25 cm high exceeds 7.7 kg, the sheets should be discarded.

7.33 Packs which are not used within one hour of preparation may be stored, providing the environmental conditions are maintained within those specified above for airing.

7.34 Non-standard test packs made of different materials (including huckaback towels TL5 or TL6 complying with BS1781) and of different sizes and weights may be used, provided they comply with BS7720. These packs may also be useful for small chambers (see paragraph 7.35).

7.35 The standard test pack should not be used where the usable chamber space is less than five times the volume of the pack. In these cases a smaller version of the pack may be constructed. This should be of cubic form with a volume about one-fifth of the usable chamber space, and made of similar materials to the standard test pack.

Use of chemical indicators

7.36 Chemical indicators are designed to show by a change of colour whether specified sterilization conditions have been attained. They should, however, always be regarded as supplementary to definitive thermometric, microbiological or (for EO) hygrometric results. Whenever a cycle variable is outside its specified limits an operating cycle should always be regarded as unsatisfactory, irrespective of the results obtained from any chemical indicators.

7.37 Chemical indicators are manufactured for a range of sterilization processes and cycle variables. They should not be used for any process other than that specified by the manufacturer. The use of an inappropriate indicator may give dangerously misleading results.

7.38 Specifications for chemical indicators for sterilization processes are given in EN 867 which is currently in preparation (1994). Two classes are applicable to the tests covered in HTM 2010.

7.39 Class A indicators ("process indicators") are intended for use with individual packs of product to demonstrate that the pack has been exposed to the sterilization process. They have a defined end-point reaction, in which a visible change occurs after exposure to the specified variables at a level equal to or greater than that specified for the indicator. Class A indicators are used alongside biological indicators in tests on LTSF and EO sterilizers to provide an early visual indication of the efficacy of gas penetration. If a chemical indicator shows a failure, then it is normal for the test to be abandoned and the cause investigated. If all chemical indicators are satisfactory, then the biological indicators should be incubated as described in the relevant test. Chemical indicators by themselves are insufficient to demonstrate the efficacy of gaseous sterilization processes. Class A indicators are specified in EN 867: Part 2.

7.40 Class B indicators are designed for use in the Bowie-Dick test for steam penetration (see paragraph 13.37). They may have either a defined end-point or a graduated response in which a progressive change occurs on exposure to one or more process variables allowing assessment of the level achieved. Class B indicators are specified in EN 867: Part 3.

7.41 Other classes of indicator are available but are not required for the tests in this HTM.

7.42 The performance of chemical indicators may be affected by the conditions of storage before use, the methods of use and the conditions of storage after exposure to the process. For these reasons the recommendations of the manufacturer for storage and use should be followed precisely. Indicators should not be used beyond any expiry date stated by the manufacturer.

Use of biological indicators

7.43 Biological indicators are designed to show by the survival of test micro-organisms whether specified sterilization conditions have been attained. The absence of growth of a test micro-organism after exposure to a sterilization process demonstrates that a specified level of microbiological inactivation has been delivered. Survival of a test micro-organism subjected to a sterilization process indicates that the process has failed. Biological indicators are required for tests on LTSF and EO sterilizers to confirm that sterilization conditions have been attained. On rare occasions they may be required for PQ tests on other types of sterilizer (see paragraph 8.9).

7.44 Terminology adopted in this HTM conforms to that given in EN 866. An **inoculated carrier** is defined as a piece of supporting material on which a defined number of test organisms has been deposited. A **biological indicator** is defined as an inoculated carrier contained within its primary pack ready for use. The relationship between the components is shown in Figure 5.

7.45 Biological indicators are manufactured for a range of sterilization processes and cycle variables. They should not be used for any process other than that specified by the manufacturer. The use of an inappropriate indicator may give dangerously misleading results.

7.46 The performance of biological indicators may be affected by the conditions of storage before use, the methods of use and the techniques employed after exposure to the process. For these reasons the recommendations of the manufacturer for storage and recovery conditions should be followed. Biological indicators should be transferred to the specified recovery conditions as soon as possible after exposure to the process and in any case within 2 hours of the end of the cycle. Indicators must not be used beyond any expiry date stated by the manufacturer.

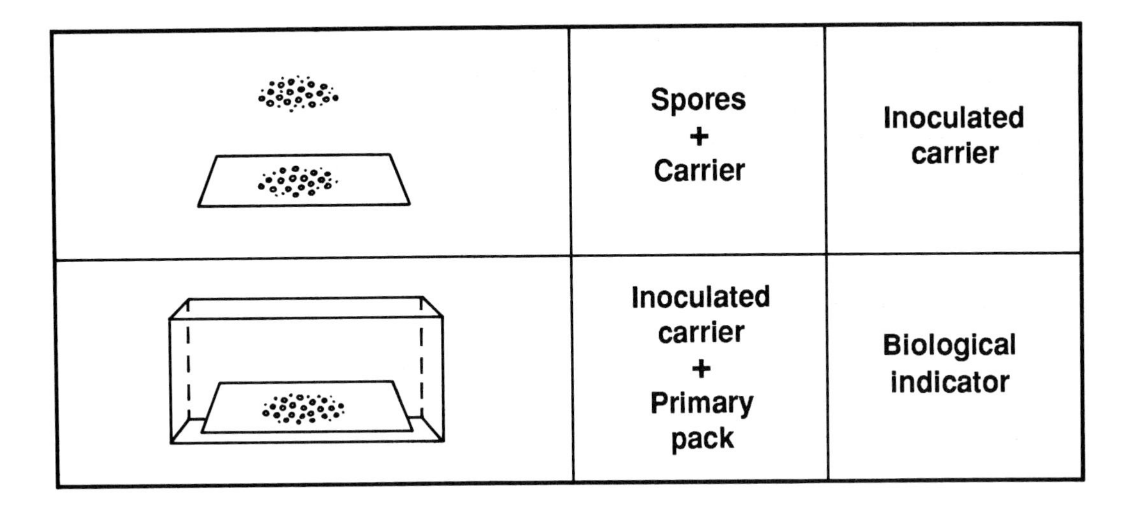

Spores
+
Carrier
Inoculated carrier
Inoculated carrier
+
Primary pack
Biological indicator

Adapted from EN 866: Part 1

Figure 5 Components of a biological indicator

7.47 Control of biological indicators should be the responsibility of the microbiologist. Incubation of indicators should be carried out by an accredited laboratory registered with CPA (UK) Ltd (see Appendix 1).

Specifications

7.48 Specifications for biological indicators for sterilization processes are given in the several Parts of EN 866, which is currently in preparation (1994). The standard draws a distinction between indicators designed for routine monitoring and indicators designed for validation tests. For routine monitoring, EN 866 specifies both the minimum number of organisms on the carrier and also a minimum D-value. For validation, no such limits are set. As a consequence, indicators manufactured in accordance with EN 866 for routine monitoring will always be suitable for validation, but the reverse will not necessarily be true.

7.49 The following organisms are recommended in EN 866 for the microbiological tests specified in this HTM. Other strains or organisms may be used provided they are demonstrated to be of equivalent performance. Addresses for culture collections may be found in Appendix 1:

a. for LTSF sterilizers, *Bacillus stearothermophilus* as specified in EN 866: Part 5. *B stearothermophilus* strains NCIMB 8224 and NCTC 10003 have been found to be suitable;

b. for EO sterilizers, *Bacillus subtilis* var *niger* as specified in EN 866: Part 2. *B subtilis* var *niger* strains ATCC 9372, CIP 7718 and NCTC 10073 have been found to be suitable.

7.50 Although not normally required for the tests in this HTM, the following organisms may be used where the need arises:

a. for high-temperature steam sterilizers, *Bacillus stearothermophilus* as specified in EN 866: Part 3. *B stearothermophilus* strains ATCC 7953, ATCC 12980, CIP 5281 and NCTC 10003 have been found to be suitable;

b. for dry-heat sterilizers, *Bacillus subtilis* as specified in EN 866: Part 6. *B subtilis* strains ATCC 9372 and CIP 7718 have been found to be suitable.

Line-Pickerell helix

7.51 The Line-Pickerell helix (Line and Pickerell, 1973) is a process challenge device used in microbiological tests on LTSF and EO sterilizers and designed to simulate the worst-case penetration conditions for sterilization by gas. The device is so constructed that an inoculated carrier can be placed within it in a position most difficult for the gas to reach.

7.52 The device consists of stainless steel tubing with a gas-tight metal capsule for the biological indicator at one end (Figure 6). The capsule is in two parts which fit together against an O-ring seal and are secured by a knurled nut. The capsule body is sealed to the stainless steel tube so that the only entry into the assembled capsule is via the whole length of the tube. The nominal dimensions of the tube are 4.55 m in length and 3.0 mm in internal diameter, presenting a single-ended system with a length-to-bore ratio of approximately 1500:1. The total internal volume of the assembly is approximately 32 ml, of which 0.85 ml comprises the capsule. For compactness, the tube is formed into a helix of nominal 115 mm diameter. The tail of the helix is turned out slightly for ease of connection to air or water services for cleaning.

7.53 Before placing an inoculated carrier in the capsule, ensure that the helix is clear by blowing oil-free compressed air through it. Check the seal for damage or deterioration. Tighten the capsule and test it for leakage by submerging the helix in water and pressurising it with oil-free air at approximately 0.15 bar.

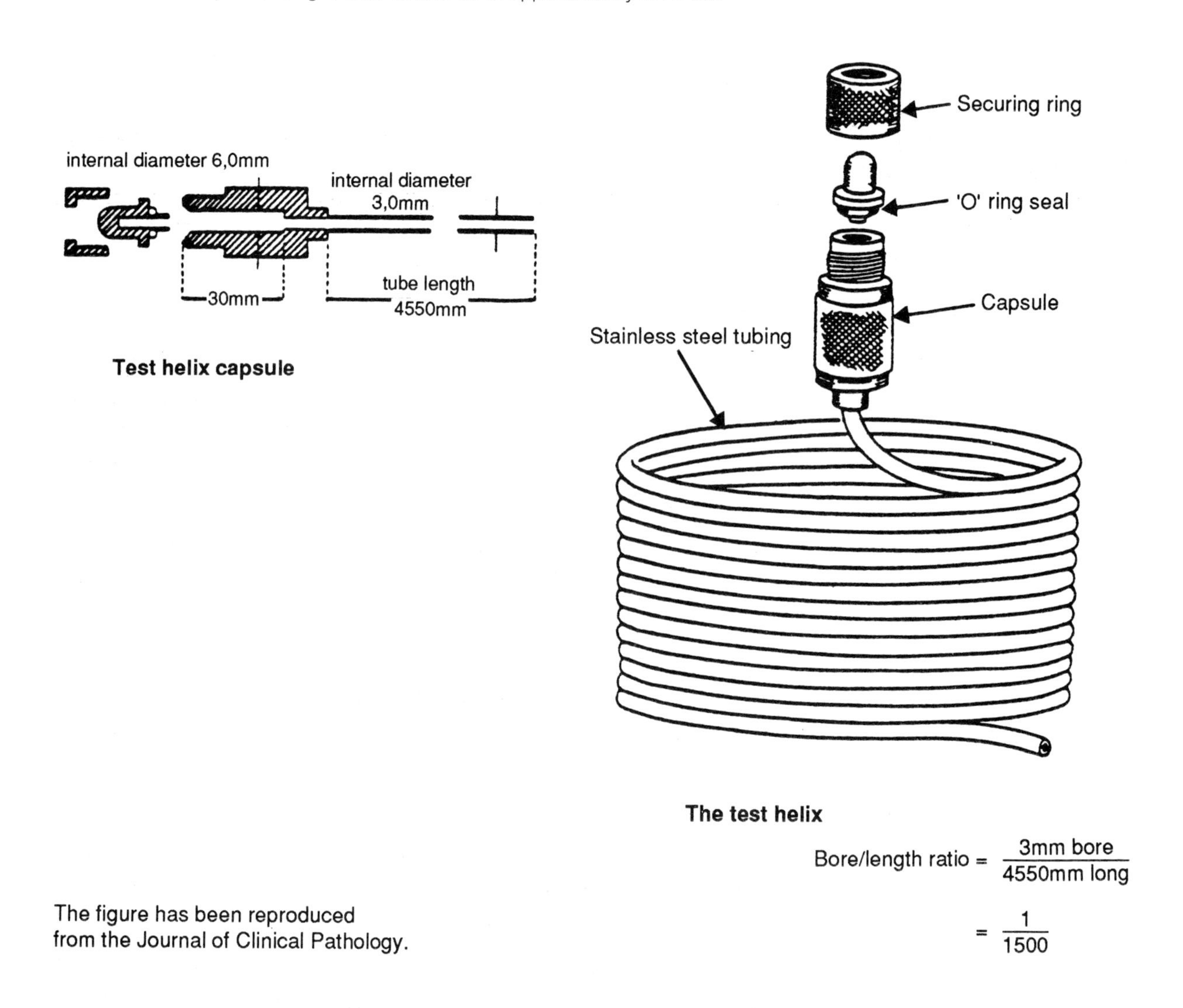

Figure 6 Line-Pickerell helix

Preparation of recovery medium

7.54 The recovery medium should be tryptone soya broth demonstrated as capable of recovering 10–100 viable spores of the test organism. Documentary evidence of performance should be provided by the manufacturer for each batch of dehydrated medium supplied.

7.55 The made-up medium should be prepared in accordance with the producer's recommendation. If no recommendation is available, proceed as follows.

7.56 Each batch should be dispensed in volumes of 15–20 ml in screw-capped bottles of at least 25 ml capacity and sterilized at a sterilization temperature of 121°C. The bottles should be stored at 2–10°C and used within 12 months.

7.57 The microbiologist should test each batch for sterility at each of the incubation temperatures at which it will be used. Select at least 2% of the bottles at random and incubate them for seven days at 52–56°C (for bottles intended for use with *B stearothermophilus*) or 30–32°C (for bottles intended for use with *B subtilis*). The batch should be considered satisfactory for use at that incubation temperature if none of the bottles shows growth. If one or more bottles does show growth, the entire batch should be regarded as not sterile.

7.58 The microbiologist should test each batch for its ability to promote growth. Test organisms which are damaged but not killed in the sterilization process may not outgrow if cultural conditions are not ideal. The following method is recommended.

Ringer's solution (full strength) is made from 9.0 g sodium chloride, 0.42 g potassium chloride, 0.48 g calcium chloride and 0.2 g sodium bicarbonate, in 1000 ml of distilled water. Source: Bacteriological tests for graded milk *(Ministry of Health, 1937).*

7.59 Remove the inoculated carriers from two biological indicators of the type to be used with the recovery medium. Place the carriers in 10 ml of quarter-strength Ringer's solution. Agitate to release the test organisms from the carriers; this may be done by ultrasonication, shaking with glass beads, or another appropriate validated method.

7.60 Dilute the solution to make a suspension with a count of 500 test organisms per ml.

7.61 Select 20 bottles at random from the sterilized batch of recovery medium. Add 0.1 ml of the suspension to each bottle. Incubate the bottles for seven days at 52–56°C (for *B stearothermophilus*) or 30–32°C (for *B subtilis*). Confirm the recovery of the test organism by subculture as described in paragraph 7.71.

7.62 The batch of recovery medium should be considered satisfactory if all 20 bottles show growth. If one or more bottles does not show growth, the entire batch should be discarded.

General procedure for microbiological tests

7.63 All biological indicators used in any one test should be taken from the same batch.

7.64 Except where specified otherwise (in certain EO tests), all the microbiological tests in this HTM require biological indicators to be used in the form of unprotected inoculated carriers without their primary packs. They should therefore be handled aseptically to avoid contamination.

7.65 Biological indicators should be positioned as described in the relevant test procedure. If chemical indicators are to be used, they should be placed alongside the biological indicators to form biological/chemical indicator pairs.

7.66 Indicators should be cultured in accordance with the manufacturer's recommendations. The use of an inappropriate recovery system can give dangerously misleading results. If no recommendation is available, proceed as follows.

7.67 Within 2 hours of the end of the cycle, aseptically transfer each inoculated carrier to a bottle of recovery medium at a temperature of 15–25°C. Fit the caps to the bottles loosely (for *B stearothermophilus*) or tightly (for *B subtilis*).

7.68 Prepare control bottles of recovery medium as follows:

a. at least three bottles (for validation tests) or at least one bottle (for periodic tests), each containing an unexposed inoculated carrier, to demonstrate that the indicators are viable;

b. at least three bottles containing recovery medium only, to demonstrate that the medium is not contaminated.

7.69 Incubate the test bottles together with the controls under the conditions shown in Table 9.

Organism	*B stearothermophilus*	*B subtilis*
Incubation temperature	52–56°C	30–32°C
Incubation time:		
for validation tests (commissioning and performance qualification)	14 days[a]	7 days
for routine tests (production cycles)	7 days	7 days

a. For validation of LTSF cycles it is recommended that biological indicators are incubated for 14 days to allow outgrowth of organisms which may have been damaged but not inactivated by exposure to the process. Once the validation tests have been successfully completed, incubation times of seven days are acceptable for subsequent routine tests.

Table 9 Recommended incubation conditions for biological indicators

7.70 Inspect the bottles periodically for signs of growth. After inspection, gently shake the bottles to aerate the medium. Control bottles should be handled in the same way as test bottles.

7.71 As soon as one or more of the test bottles becomes turbid, confirm the isolation of the test organism as follows. Take a sample from each turbid test bottle and from each positive control bottle and streak them on to tryptone soya agar on vented plates. *B stearothermophilus* should be incubated at 52–56°C in an airtight container (such as a plastic bag) to prevent the agar drying out. *B subtilis* should be incubated at 30–32°C. If there is no growth on the test plates after 18–24 hours, the cloudiness is not due to microbial growth. The positive control plate should show characteristic colonies of the test organism as described in *A colour atlas of Bacillus species* (Parry, Turnbull and Gibson, 1983).

7.72 The test should be considered satisfactory if the following requirements are met:

a. chemical indicators show a uniform colour change at the end of the cycle;

b. all bottles containing an inoculated carrier exposed to the sterilization process show no growth at the end of the incubation time;

c. all control bottles containing an unexposed inoculated carrier show growth of the test organism within 24 hours;

d. all control bottles without an inoculated carrier show no growth at the end of the incubation time.

7.73 All culture results should be noted, whether satisfactory or not.

7.74 Where growth has resulted from an organism other than the test organism, the test is inconclusive and should be repeated.

7.75 Note the following:

a. as a rough guide, the earlier the growth appears during the incubation period, the less efficacious is the sterilization process;

b. consistent failures in one position in the chamber may indicate problems of gas distribution (for example, stratification);

c. failure in a helix with no failures in the chamber free space may indicate poor gas penetration possibly due to inadequate air removal, excessively wet steam, or (for EO) low humidity;

d. for LTSF sterilizers, failure in the chamber with no failure in a helix may indicate low humidity due to the chamber wall being too hot or the steam being superheated.

8.0 Performance qualification

Introduction

8.1 Performance qualification (PQ) is defined as the process of obtaining and documenting evidence that the sterilizer, as commissioned, will produce acceptable goods when operated in accordance with the operational instructions. PQ tests are performed as part of the initial validation procedure, as part of any repeat validation procedure, and whenever the user judges that a new loading condition calls for a new PQ test.

8.2 Performance qualification should not be attempted on any sterilizer that fails to meet the requirements of the commissioning tests specified in Chapters 4 and 5.

8.3 Thermometric PQ is required for all sterilizers. Additional microbiological PQ tests, and PQ tests for environmental gas and load degassing times, are required for LTSF and EO sterilizers.

8.4 Information gathered from the PQ test is filed in a PQ report which specifies the standard of performance expected with a particular operating cycle and loading condition (see paragraph 8.7). The report includes a master process record, employed by the user to validate routine production loads, together with thermometric and (where required) microbiological data used for subsequent performance requalification.

8.5 Performance requalification (PRQ) is the process of confirming that the sterilizer continues to meet the performance standards established during performance qualification, and that the working data collected during performance qualification remain valid. It is carried out once a year as part of the yearly test schedule, as part of any revalidation process, or whenever the user requests such confirmation.

8.6 PQ and PRQ tests should normally be preceded by the basic performance tests specified in the commissioning and yearly test schedules.

Loading conditions and reference loads

8.7 A **loading condition** is a specified combination of the nature and number of load items, the items of chamber furniture, and their distribution within the chamber. For example, a load placed on the top shelf of the chamber constitutes a different loading condition from an identical load placed on the bottom shelf. In principle, validation is not complete until a PQ test has been performed for each loading condition that the sterilizer is expected to process. In practice, loading conditions specified in the thermometric tests for small and full loads carried out during commissioning are designed to be representative of the nature of production loads, and to present a greater challenge to the process than most production loads. In these cases PQ data may be taken from the commissioning tests and PQ tests may not be necessary.

8.8 Guidance on the design of loading conditions to achieve efficient sterilization can be found in Part 4 of this HTM.

8.9 PQ tests are indicated in the following circumstances:

a. where the loading condition presents a greater challenge to the process than that presented by the commissioning tests. For example, while porous load sterilizers rarely need PQ tests, such tests will be required if the density of the porous material exceeds that of the standard test pack (see paragraph 7.27) or if narrow lumens restrict air removal and steam penetration;

b. where the nature of the load is not represented by the commissioning tests. For example, certain loads may be damaged by exposure to the normal sterilization temperature. In these cases, the settings of cycle variables and their permitted tolerances should ensure not only that the load is sterilized, but also that it is not unacceptably degraded by long exposure to high temperatures.

8.10 Where PQ tests are required it is often possible to select a production load that is known to present a greater challenge to the process than any of the others. This **reference load** can then serve as a worst case and allow one PQ test to be valid for a range of less demanding loading conditions.

8.11 A microbiological PQ test is required for LTSF and EO sterilizers in addition to the thermometric test. It may also be required for other sterilizers where air removal and steam penetration are difficult, and a thermometric test does not provide sufficient assurance that the sterilization conditions have been attained throughout the load.

8.12 Responsibility for deciding which loading conditions require PQ tests is exercised as follows (in doubtful cases advice should be sought from the authorised person:

a. sterilizers to be used for medicinal products – jointly by the user, the quality controller and the test person;

b. LTSF and EO sterilizers – jointly by the user, the microbiologist and the test person;

c. all other sterilizers – jointly by the user and the test person.

Thermometric test for performance qualification

8.13 This test is suitable for all steam sterilizers, that is, porous loads, fluids, unwrapped instruments and utensils, LTS, LTSF and laboratory sterilizers. (See Chapter 16 for dry-heat sterilizers, and Chapter 18 for EO sterilizers.)

8.14 The production load under test will normally consist of discrete items such as packs, bottles or other containers. Place temperature sensors in the following positions:

a. one in each of three items known to be the slowest to attain the sterilization temperature;

b. one in each of three items known to be the fastest to attain the sterilization temperature;

c. if the sterilizer has a thermal door interlock, one in each of three items known to be the slowest to cool to 80°C.

8.15 If the load consists of less than six items, then place a sensor in each item.

8.16 The sensors should be in good thermal contact with the fluid or device which they are monitoring, and placed, if possible, in or on the part of the item slowest to heat up. (See Chapter 6 for guidance on the use of temperature sensors.)

8.17 The fastest and slowest items should have been identified as part of the design of the loading condition as described in Part 4. It may be desirable to confirm that the correct items have been selected by placing additional sensors in neighbouring items and running one or more preliminary operating cycles to verify that the selected items are indeed the fastest and slowest.

8.18 Place a sensor either in an active chamber discharge (see paragraph 6.26) or in the coolest part of the chamber. (This will normally be close to the sensor connected to the sterilizer recording instrument.)

8.19 Insert any load temperature probes provided in the chamber into the positions they will normally occupy in the load. If a probe is required to occupy the same position as a sensor, then the sensor should be moved to a neighbouring load item if they cannot both be accommodated in the same load item.

8.20 Note the loading condition and the positions of the sensors and probes in sufficient detail for the test to be replicated on any future occasion.

8.21 If the sterilizer has a pressure instrument, connect a pressure recorder (or test gauge) to the chamber.

8.22 Select the operating cycle that will be used for the production load. Start the cycle.

8.23 Ensure that a batch process record is made by the recording instrument fitted to the sterilizer. This will serve as the basis for a master process record for the loading condition under test (see paragraph 8.58). If the sterilizer does not have a recorder (such as some machines for unwrapped instruments and utensils), note the elapsed time, indicated chamber temperatures and pressures at all significant points of the operating cycle, for example the beginning and end of each stage or sub-stage.

8.24 At the approximate mid-point of the plateau period, note the elapsed time and indicated chamber temperature and pressure.

8.25 For fluid loads, during the cooling stage wait for the temperature in the containers to fall to 95°C (plastic containers) or 85°C (glass). Wearing protective visor and gloves, attempt to open the door. As soon as the cycle is complete, but before opening the door, note the recorded temperature in the containers.

8.26 The test should be considered satisfactory if the following requirements are met:

a. the requirements of the automatic control test (see paragraph 12.13) are met;

b. the holding time, as determined from the measured temperatures, is not less than that specified for the appropriate sterilization temperature band in Table 8;

c. during the holding time:

   (i) the measured temperatures are within the sterilization temperature band specified for the operating cycle;

   (ii) the indicated and recorded chamber temperatures are within 2°C of the temperature measured in the active chamber discharge;

(iii) the temperature measured in each load item does not fluctuate more than ± 1°C, and does not differ from that in other load items by more than 2°C;

(iv) the indicated and recorded chamber pressures are within 0.05 bar of the measured pressure;

d. at the end of the cycle:

(i) the temperature sensors have remained in position;

(ii) the items containing sensors are intact;

(iii) the temperature measured in any fluid containers is not greater than 90°C (plastic) or 80°C (glass).

8.27 If the test is satisfactory, it should be performed two more times to check for reproducibility and to establish permitted tolerances (see paragraph 8.47). A master process record should then be made as described below (see paragraph 8.58).

8.28 If, having completed the commissioning tests, the sterilizer fails to meet the above requirements then it is possible that the sterilizer is not capable of processing the load. Advice should be sought from the authorised person.

Microbiological test for performance qualification

8.29 This test is designed to be used in exceptional circumstances as an additional PQ test for steam and dry-heat sterilizers. (See Chapter 17 for LTSF sterilizers, and Chapter 18 for EO sterilizers.)

8.30 The microbiological test should follow a satisfactory thermometric test, and use the identical loading condition and operating cycle. (See Chapter 7 for information on the use of biological and chemical indicators.)

8.31 Put a biological indicator and a chemical indicator together in each of the six load items that carried temperature sensors in the thermometric test. Place the items in as nearly as possible the same positions they occupied in the thermometric test.

8.32 Select and start the operating cycle.

8.33 Ensure that a batch process record is made by the recording instrument fitted to the sterilizer. If the sterilizer does not have a recorder (such as some machines for unwrapped instruments and utensils), observe and note the elapsed time, indicated chamber temperatures and pressures at all significant points of the operating cycle, for example the beginning and end of each stage or sub-stage.

8.34 At the approximate mid-point of the plateau period, note the elapsed time and indicated chamber temperature and pressure.

8.35 At the end of the cycle, remove the indicators from the load items. Check that the chemical indicators show a uniform colour change. If so, place each of the inoculated carriers in a bottle of recovery medium and incubate them with controls as described in the general procedure for microbiological tests (see paragraphs 7.63–75).

8.36 The test should be considered satisfactory if the following requirements are met:

a. during the whole of the cycle the values of the cycle variables as shown on the batch process record are within the permitted tolerances marked on the master process record established during the thermometric PQ test;

b. the requirements for microbiological tests set out in paragraph 7.72 are met.

Environmental gas test

8.37 This PQ test is designed to determine the concentration of formaldehyde or EO gas discharged into the loading area from the chamber and load at the end of a cycle. The concentration will vary with the type of load, wrapping material and environmental ventilation and temperature.

8.38 This test should follow a satisfactory thermometric PQ test. The loading condition, preconditioning process and operating cycle should be identical. The test may be combined with the microbiological PQ test.

8.39 A gas monitoring instrument as described in Chapter 6 is required.

8.40 Load the chamber as for the microbiological test for performance qualification.

8.41 Select the operating cycle used in the microbiological test. Start the cycle.

8.42 At the end of the cycle, measure the concentration of gas discharged from the chamber into the air when the door starts to open. The sample should be taken 80–120 mm in front of the gap at a height of 1.4–1.6 m. Continue to monitor the gas concentration for the next 15 min.

8.43 Determine the average concentration of gas over the 15-min period.

8.44 The test should be considered satisfactory if the average concentration of gas over the 15-min period does not exceed the short-term exposure limit specified in Table 1.

8.45 The data from the test should be used to establish a permitted upper limit for subsequent performance requalification. This should be as low as reasonably practicable, and in any case lower than the short-term exposure limit (see paragraph 1.28).

Test for degassing time

8.46 Loads from LTSF and EO sterilizers require a further PQ test to determine the minimum degassing time required before a load may be released for clinical use. It is the responsibility of the user to establish this period for the area in which sterilized loads are stored. Procedures for determining the levels of residual EO are described in EN 30993: Part 7; a standard for formaldehyde is under development.

Permitted tolerances

8.47 It is the purpose of performance qualification to establish the standard of performance expected with a particular operating cycle and loading condition, so that subsequent production cycles can be judged by that standard. The evidence for this performance is provided by the indicated, recorded and measured cycle variables, and it is necessary to determine how much each variable will be permitted to vary from cycle to cycle while still conforming to that standard.

8.48 A starting point is the limits prescribed for the cycle variables in the commissioning and PQ tests described in this HTM. Other than in exceptional circumstances, these limits should be regarded as absolute, and a failure to meet them implies a failure of the test and a gross failure of the sterilizer. These limits originate from European and British Standards and from operational experience. They are set to accommodate a wide range of sterilizer models and designs of operating cycles. However, an individual sterilizer should be able to repeat a cycle well within these limits, and the permitted tolerances for PQ purposes should be correspondingly smaller.

8.49 It is important that the tolerances are set with careful consideration of the likely range of variation from cycle to cycle. If set too tight, acceptable production loads may be erroneously rejected as non-sterile, and automatic control and PRQ tests may fail unnecessarily. However, it would be a mistake to set an over-generous tolerance, since that may disguise variations signalling a developing malfunction of the sterilizer. The following paragraphs give guidance on determining the permitted tolerances. The authorised person should be consulted in cases of doubt.

8.50 PQ tests (or commissioning tests providing PQ data) collect indicated, recorded and measured data (see paragraph 7.2–7.20 for an explanation of these terms). The three sets of data serve different purposes and may require different tolerances:

a. **indicated data** are available to the user for production cycles on all types of sterilizer, but cannot be regarded as definitive. Except for sterilizers without a recorder, PQ tests require indicated values to be noted only during the holding time to ensure that they comply with the sterilization conditions;

b. **recorded data** are available to the user for production cycles on most types of sterilizer and can be regarded as definitive for routine production control. The permitted tolerances are normally marked on a master process record (see paragraph 8.58). The user should be aware of any calibration error in the recorder, but since production cycles are validated by direct comparison of the batch process record (BPR) with the master process record (MPR), such errors can be ignored in determining the permitted tolerances;

c. **measured data** are not available for production cycles and so play no part in routine monitoring. However, they are to be regarded as definitive for the purposes of performance requalification. Measured variables are more reliable than indicated or recorded values, and the permitted tolerances should reflect this.

8.51 A further consideration is the intended use of the PQ data:

a. **PQ data valid for a single loading condition**: where the PQ data are to be used for one loading condition only, the variation between cycles is essentially random (that is, due to uncontrolled variables or the intrinsic performance limits of the sterilizer) and the permitted tolerances can be tight. This is appropriate, as such cases are often used for loads which would be damaged if the limits were broader. The tolerances should be set by experience of the sterilizer and of the cycle. The three replicate thermometric PQ tests (see paragraph 8.13) will give some indication of what variation to expect;

b. **PQ data valid for a range of loading conditions**: where the PQ data for a single loading condition is judged to be valid for a range of loading conditions, the variation between cycles will contain a systematic variation related to the differing loading conditions and therefore the permitted tolerances will be greater. The choice of loading conditions for which the data is valid should take into account whether this greater tolerance is acceptable;

c. **PQ data obtained from commissioning tests**: for many loads, especially on porous load sterilizers, PQ tests are not normally necessary and data from the thermometric commissioning tests are used to establish performance standards for a wide range of loading conditions. In these cases, data from the small-load and full-load tests can be used to establish the limits of variation for production loads which fall between these two extremes. The permitted tolerances will be broader than either (a) or (b).

8.52 Note that the permitted tolerances during the holding time of an operating cycle will generally be tighter than those allowed during the preceding and following stages. In no circumstances should these tolerances permit the cycle variables to depart from the sterilization conditions specified in Table 8, unless the operating cycle has been designed with that intention.

8.53 Tolerances are normally expressed as a permitted variation either side of a central value, either in absolute terms or as a percentage. In some cases the tolerances may be expressed as an upper or lower limit, with the variables permitted to take any value on the "safe" side of the limit.

PQ report

8.54 All the data collected during PQ tests should be filed in a PQ report, a copy of which should be kept with the plant history file. The report should contain or refer to the complete specification for the sterilization process. The specification should be detailed enough to allow the loading condition, the operating cycle and the test itself to be replicated on any future occasion. The report should include the following:

a. a specification of the loading condition, defined either by the nature and number of load items, items of chamber furniture, and their distribution within the chamber, or by a coded reference to a detailed specification held elsewhere;

b. a specification of the operating cycle, defined either by the settings for the cycle variables or by a coded reference to a detailed specification held elsewhere;

c. a specification of any preconditioning, conditioning and degassing process (this is essential for EO sterilizers);

d. all the indicated, recorded and measured data from the test, drawing attention to the values and permitted tolerances of elapsed time and of the indicated, recorded and measured cycle variables at all significant points of the operating cycle, for example at the beginning and end of each stage or sub-stage (the tolerances in recorded variables should also be marked on the master process record);

e. for loads which require the removal of air before sterilization, the method used to verify whether the minimum conditions of steam penetration into the load are attained (for porous load sterilizers, this is by use of the air detector);

f. the original of the master process record derived from the test.

8.55 EO sterilizers require extensive additional data for safety and quality control purposes and these are listed in Table 11.

8.56 Immediately following the PQ tests, the test person should prepare PQ summary sheets (see Appendix 3) and working copies of any necessary master process records. These should be given to the user and kept with the sterilizer process log.

8.57 If PQ tests are not required, the PQ summary sheet should contain data from the thermometric test for a full load and be marked accordingly.

Preparation of a master process record

8.58 A master process record (MPR) is a record of the values and permitted tolerances of cycle variables for a correctly functioning operating cycle against which test and production cycles can be checked. (The term "master temperature record" was used in previous editions of HTM 10.) It is derived either from the batch process record (BPR) obtained during a thermometric PQ test or, if no PQ test has been deemed necessary, from the BPR obtained from a full-load thermometric test carried out during commissioning. (A further MPR may be required to validate automatic control tests with an empty chamber.) It may be a one-to-one transparent copy of the BPR, a "template" derived from the BPR, or data stored in a computer control system and compared automatically.

8.59 An MPR is primarily intended for production control on sterilizers used to process medicinal products, but it is also used for test purposes on all types of sterilizer.

8.60 When required for production purposes, a sufficient number and variety of MPRs should be prepared so that there is a suitable MPR for each loading condition or for the appropriate reference load (see paragraph 8.10).

8.61 To prepare an MPR, the appropriate thermometric test should be carried out as described above (see paragraph 8.13). If all three cycles are satisfactory, the BPR showing the shortest holding time should be used for producing the MPR. It should be marked with the following information:

a. an MPR reference number and reference to the PQ report;

b. sufficient information to identify the sterilizer uniquely (by a unique reference number; by the name of the manufacturer, the model of sterilizer and the serial number; or by any sufficient combination of these);

c. a specification of the loading condition as in paragraph 8.54a and other loading conditions for which the MPR is valid;

d. a specification of the operating cycle as in paragraph 8.54b;

e. the permitted tolerances for the cycle variables during each stage of the operating cycle (these are best shown graphically);

f. for fluid loads, the point during the cycle at which the temperature of the fluid in the hottest container falls to 80°C (glass) or 90°C (plastic);

g. date of test;

h. signatures of the test person and the user.

8.62 When the BPR has been annotated it may be endorsed "master process record" and a transparency obtained. An example of an MPR is shown in Figure 7.

8.63 If the BPR is in the form of numerical data, the MPR should be presented in a similar form to the BPR to permit ready comparison. As a minimum

Reference
15-26-03-85

Site & Dept.
Western General
Pharmacy

P.Q. report reference
SDE/3/X

Make of sterilizer
& serial number
DAB – FC/378/93

Type of sterilizer
Fluid Mk4
RCF

Loading condition
reference
P/326

Location of load
temperature probe
Lower front centre

Operating cycle
reference
OC/31

Chart Speed
1cm = 2 minutes

Test Person
J Stern
26 January 1993

User
T Pear
26 January 1993

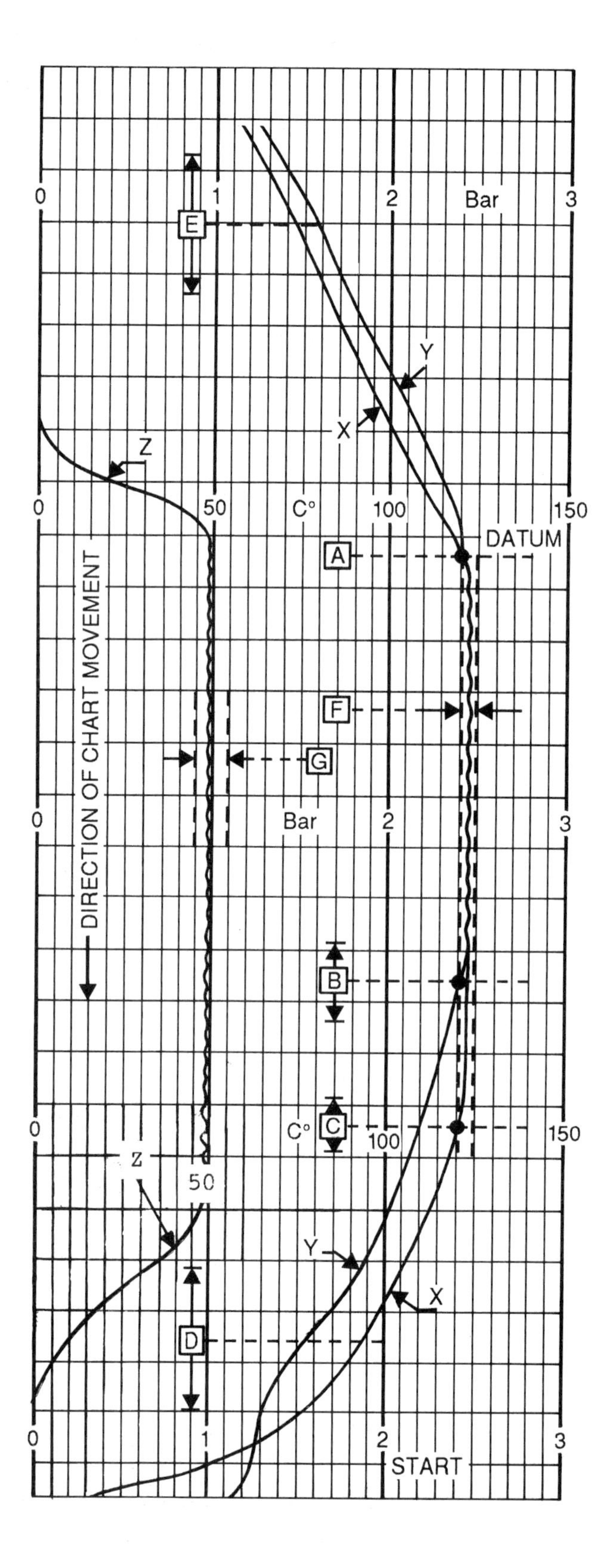

Figure 7 Example of Master Process Record (analogue)

Reference - *15-26-03-85*

Site and department - *Western General/Pharmacy*

PQ report reference - *SDE/3/X*

Make of sterilizer and serial number - *DAB FC/378/93*

Type of sterilizer - *Fluid Mk4 RCF*

Loading condition reference - *P/326*

Location of load temperature probe - *Lower front centre*

Operating cycle reference - *OC/31*

Sterilization temperature - *121°C*

Sterilization temperature band (F) - *3°C*

Sterilization pressure band - *0.15 bar*

Holding time - *15 Minutes*

Stage		Time	Temperature °C		Pressure	F (O)
		min/sec	Drain	Load	m bar	min
Heating		0.00	22.2	20.0	996	0.0
	(D)	5.15	110.0	80.1	1450	0.0
	(C)	14.45	121.1	110.2	2060	0.0
Holding Time	(B)					
		21.15	122.1	121.1	2155	5.6
		22.00	122.1	121.2	2161	6.5
		22.45	122.1	121.4	2165	7.2
		23.30	122.1	121.5	2163	6.6
		24.15	122.3	121.7	2163	8.9
		25.00	122.1	121.7	2177	9.8
		23.45	122.3	121.8	2147	10.6
		26.30	122.3	121.9	2167	11.5
		27.15	122.3	121.9	2187	12.4
		28.00	122.3	122.1	2160	13.4
		28.45	122.4	122.1	2171	14.2
		29.30	122.3	122.0	2173	15.2
		30.15	122.3	122.1	2182	16.2
		31.00	122.4	122.1	2162	17.2
		31.45	122.4	122.1	2151	18.0
		32.30	122.4	122.1	2166	18.9
		33.15	122.4	122.1	2166	19.8
		34.00	122.4	122.2	2171	20.9
		34.45	122.4	122.2	2151	21.8
		35.30	122.4	122.2	2153	22.7
		36.15	122.5	122.3	2156	23.7
	(A)	37.00	115.6	121.0	2260	24.2
Cooling		37.45	113.6	120.1	2270	24.4
	(E)	98.15	39.2	80.0	2271	24.8
		101.00	35.4	76.3	2216	24.8
		103.15	31.1	75.2	846	24.8
Venting		104.00	31.1	75.2	846	24.8
		104.45	26.1	74.8	995	24.8
End		-	-	-	-	-

Test Person J Stern Date: 26 January 1993
User T Pear Date: 26 January 1993

Figure 8 Example of Master Process Record (digital)

requirement, it should list the cycle variables at each turning point of the cycle and contain a plot generated from the data. An example of a digital MPR is shown in Figure 8.

Tests for performance requalification

8.64 PRQ tests are performed once a year to ensure that the sterilization conditions are still met. They should follow the yearly schedule of checks and tests listed in Chapter 5. For a given operating cycle it is normally necessary only to perform the PRQ test for a reference load for which a PQ report exists. The cycle can then be assumed to be effective for less demanding loads also. The need for PRQ tests on other loads should be agreed between the user and the test person.

8.65 The procedure for the PRQ test is similar to that for the PQ test. The operating cycle and the loading condition should be identical to those used for the original PQ test. The test should be considered satisfactory if the values of the measured cycle variables are within the tolerances stated in the PQ report.

8.66 For dry-heat sterilizers, fluid sterilizers and certain fluid cycles on laboratory sterilizers, a simplified PRQ test is required at quarterly intervals, and this is provided for in the schedules (see Tables 4 and 5).

8.67 Results of PRQ tests should be appended to the relevant PQ report.

8.68 Providing the yearly test programme has been completed satisfactorily, the sterilizer should pass the PRQ test. If the PRQ test is not satisfactory, the advice of the authorised person should be sought.

Notes to Figures 7 and 8

Figure 7 shows a typical master process record (MPR) for a fluid sterilizer. This is based on a batch process record made during a performance qualification test at a sterilization temperature of 121°C.

X Temperature recorded in the active chamber discharge.

Y Temperature recorded in the load item slowest to attain the sterilization temperature.

Z Chamber pressure.

A The end of the holding time is taken as the datum point from which intervals are measured.

B Start of the holding time, with permitted tolerance.

C Start of the plateau period, with permitted tolerance.

D Temperature in the load item attains 80°C.

E Temperature in the load item falls to 80°C. The door may be opened at this point.

F Sterilization temperature band.

G Sterilization pressure, with permitted tolerance.

The following deviations from the MPR are considered acceptable:

interval A–B, ± 10%;

interval A–C, ± 10%;

interval A–E, ± 20%;

interval B–D, ± 20%.

9.0 Steam quality tests

Introduction

9.1 A continuous supply of saturated steam is required for steam sterilization and for humidification in certain EO sterilizers. Too high a level of non-condensable gases will prevent the attainment of sterilizing conditions; too little moisture carried in suspension may allow the steam to become superheated during expansion into the chamber, while excess moisture may cause damp loads.

9.2 For all these tests, the steam should be sampled from the steam service pipe to each sterilizer. The measurements are taken during a period of maximum steam demand, when steam is first admitted to the sterilizer chamber.

9.3 Silicone rubber tubing is porous to steam and should not be used to carry steam in these tests.

Non-condensable gas test

9.4 This test is used to demonstrate that the level of non-condensable gases in the steam will not prevent the attainment of sterilization conditions in any part of the load. (Possible sources of non-condensable gases are discussed in Part 2 of this HTM.) The method described should be regarded not as measuring the exact level of non-condensable gas, but a method by which the provision of acceptable steam quality can be demonstrated.

9.5 The apparatus is shown and described in Figure 9. All sizes are nominal.

9.6 Connect the needle valve to the steam service pipe as shown in Figure 9.

9.7 Assemble the apparatus so that condensate will drain freely from the long rubber tube into the sampling pipe. If the tube is too short, copper or stainless steel tubing may also be used.

9.8 Fill the container with cold water until it overflows. Fill the burette and funnel with cold water, invert them and place them in the container. Draw out any air that has collected in the burette.

9.9 With the steam sampling pipe out of the container, open the needle valve and allow steam to purge the air from the pipe. Place the pipe in the container, locate the end within the funnel, and add more cold water until it flows through the overflow pipe.

9.10 Place the empty measuring cylinder under the container overflow.

9.11 Adjust the needle valve to allow a continuous sample of steam into the funnel sufficient to cause a small amount of "steam hammer" to be heard. Ensure that all the steam is discharged into the funnel and does not bubble out into the container. Note the setting of the needle valve. Close the valve.

9.12 Ensure that the container is topped up with cold water and that the measuring cylinder is empty. Draw out any air present in the burette.

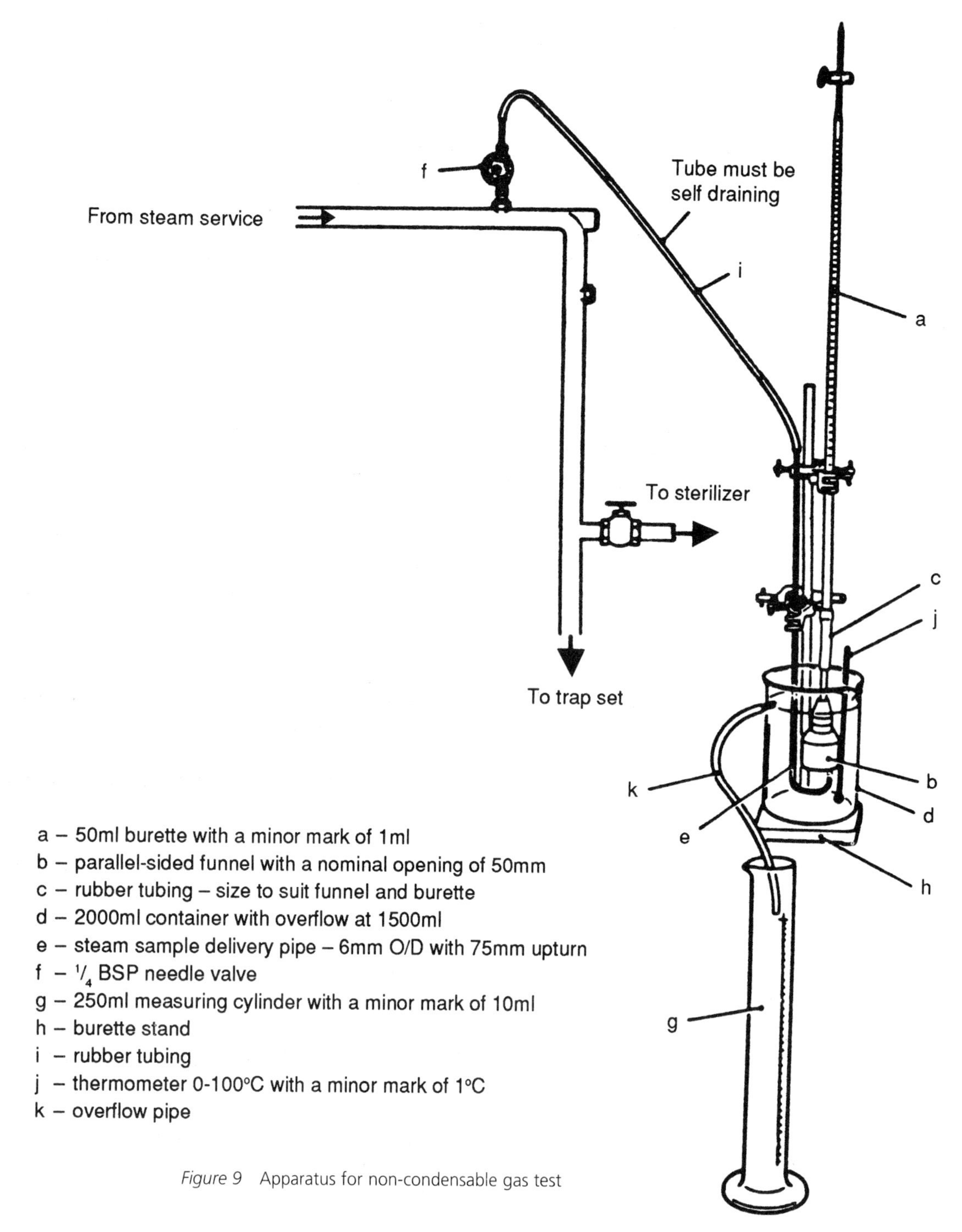

Figure 9 Apparatus for non-condensable gas test

9.13 Ensure that the sterilizer chamber is empty except for the usual chamber furniture. Select and start the operating cycle.

9.14 When the steam supply to the chamber first opens, open the needle valve to the previously noted setting, allowing a continuous sample of steam into the funnel sufficient to cause a small amount of steam hammer to be heard.

9.15 Allow the steam sample to condense in the funnel. Any non-condensable gases will rise to the top of the burette. Overspill formed by the condensate and the water displaced by the gases will collect in the measuring cylinder.

9.16 When the temperature of the water in the container reaches 70–75°C, close the needle valve. Note the volume of gas collected in the burette (V_b) and the volume of water collected in the measuring cylinder (V_c).

9.17 Calculate the fraction of non-condensable gases as a percentage as follows:

Fraction of non-condensable gases = 100 × (V_b/V_c).

9.18 The test should be considered satisfactory if the fraction of non-condensable gases does not exceed 3.5%.

9.19 The test should be done two more times to check consistency. If the results of the three tests differ significantly, then the cause should be investigated before proceeding further.

Superheat test

9.20 This test is used to demonstrate that the amount of moisture in suspension with steam from the service supply is sufficient to prevent the steam from becoming superheated during expansion into the chamber.

9.21 The method described here uses a low-volume sample, continuously taken from the centre of the steam service pipe. The level of superheat determined by this method cannot be regarded as indicative of the true dryness of the steam in the pipe since condensate flowing along the inner surface is not collected. However, devices designed to separate free condensate are incorporated into the steam delivery system to the chamber and therefore the level determined by this method is representative of steam conditions likely to prevail within the chamber during the plateau period.

9.22 This test should normally follow a satisfactory test for non-condensable gases.

9.23 This test, and the subsequent dryness value test, require a pitot tube as shown in Figure 10. The rest of the apparatus is shown and described in Figure 11. All sizes are nominal.

9.24 Fit the pitot tube concentrically within the steam service pipe as shown in Figure 11.

9.25 Fit the sensor entry gland to the steam service pipe. Insert one of the sensors through the gland and position it on the axis of the pipe.

9.26 Insert the second sensor through the gland in the expansion tube and position it on the axis of the pipe. Wrap lagging around the expansion tube. Push the tube on to the pitot.

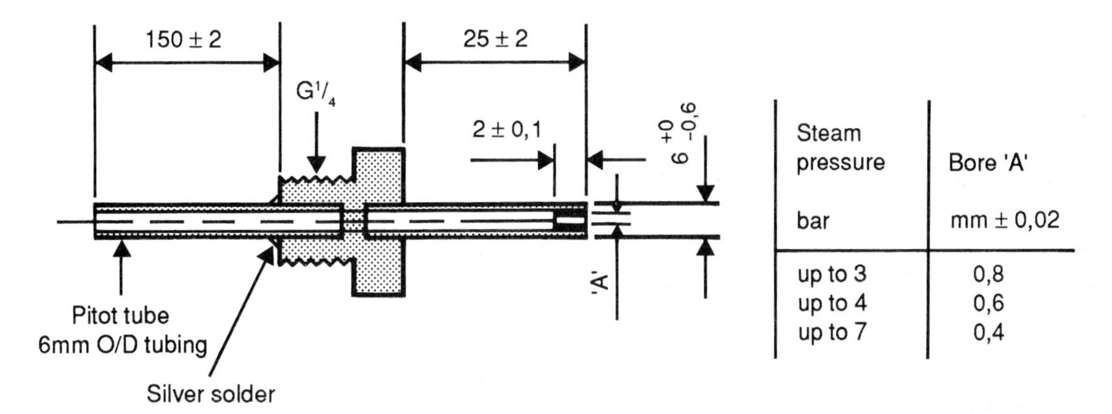

Steam pressure bar	Bore 'A' mm ± 0,02
up to 3	0,8
up to 4	0,6
up to 7	0,4

Figure 10 Pitot tube

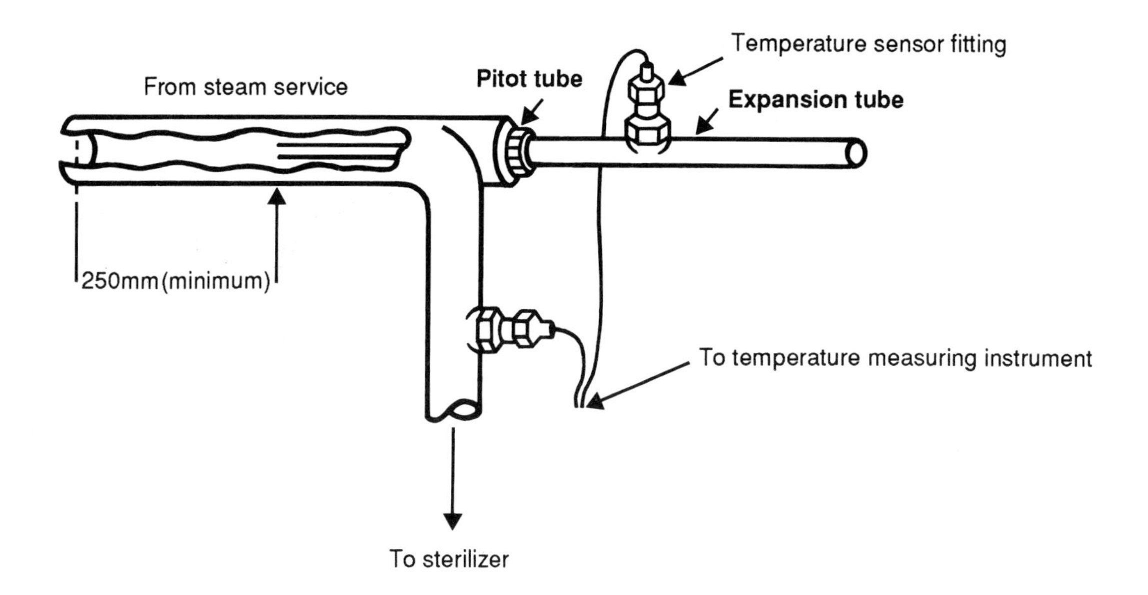

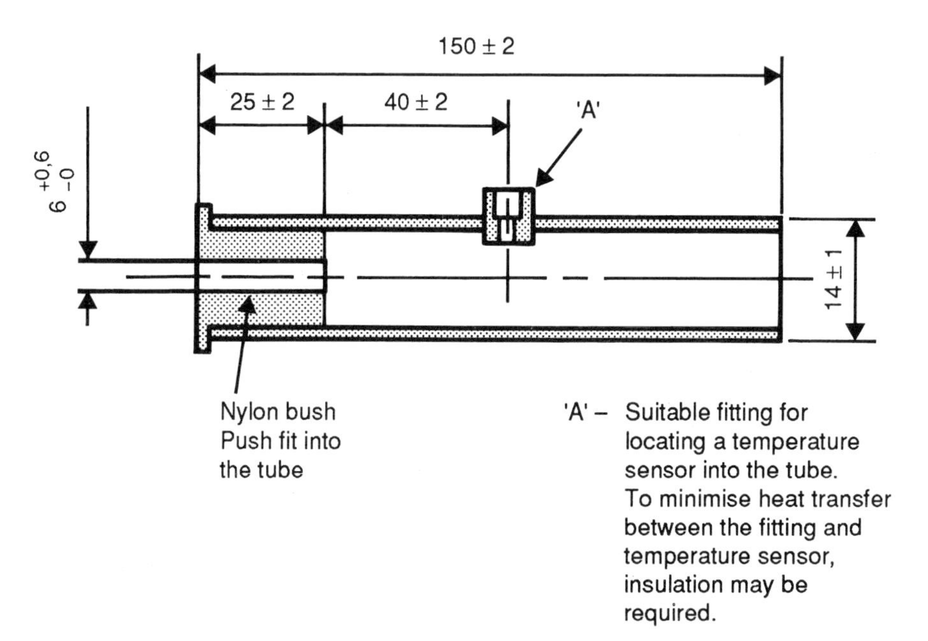

Figure 11 Apparatus for superheat test

9.27 Ensure that the sterilizer chamber is empty except for the usual chamber furniture. Select and start the operating cycle.

9.28 From the measured temperatures, note the temperature in the steam service pipe (for use in the dryness test) and in the expansion tube (T_e) when the steam supply to the chamber first opens. Calculate the superheat in °C from the following equation:

Superheat = $T_e - T_0$

where T_0 is the boiling point of water at local atmospheric pressure.

9.29 The test should be considered satisfactory if the superheat measured in the expansion tube does not exceed 25°C.

Dryness test

9.30 The accurate measurement of the percentage of moisture content in the steam is difficult, and the traditional methods where constant steam flow is required are not suitable for sterilizers. This test should be regarded not as measuring the true content of moisture in the steam, but as a method by which the provision of acceptable steam quality can be demonstrated. Possible sources of excess moisture are discussed in Part 2 of this HTM.

9.31 The test is conveniently carried out immediately after the superheat test.

9.32 This test requires a pitot tube as shown in Figure 10. The apparatus is shown and described in Figure 12. All sizes are nominal. A laboratory balance is also required, capable of weighing a load up to 2 kg with an accuracy of 0.1 g or better.

9.33 If it is not already fitted, fit the pitot tube concentrically within the steam service pipe as shown in Figure 12.

9.34 If it is not already fitted, fit the sensor entry gland to the steam service pipe. Insert a temperature sensor through the gland and position it on the axis of the pipe.

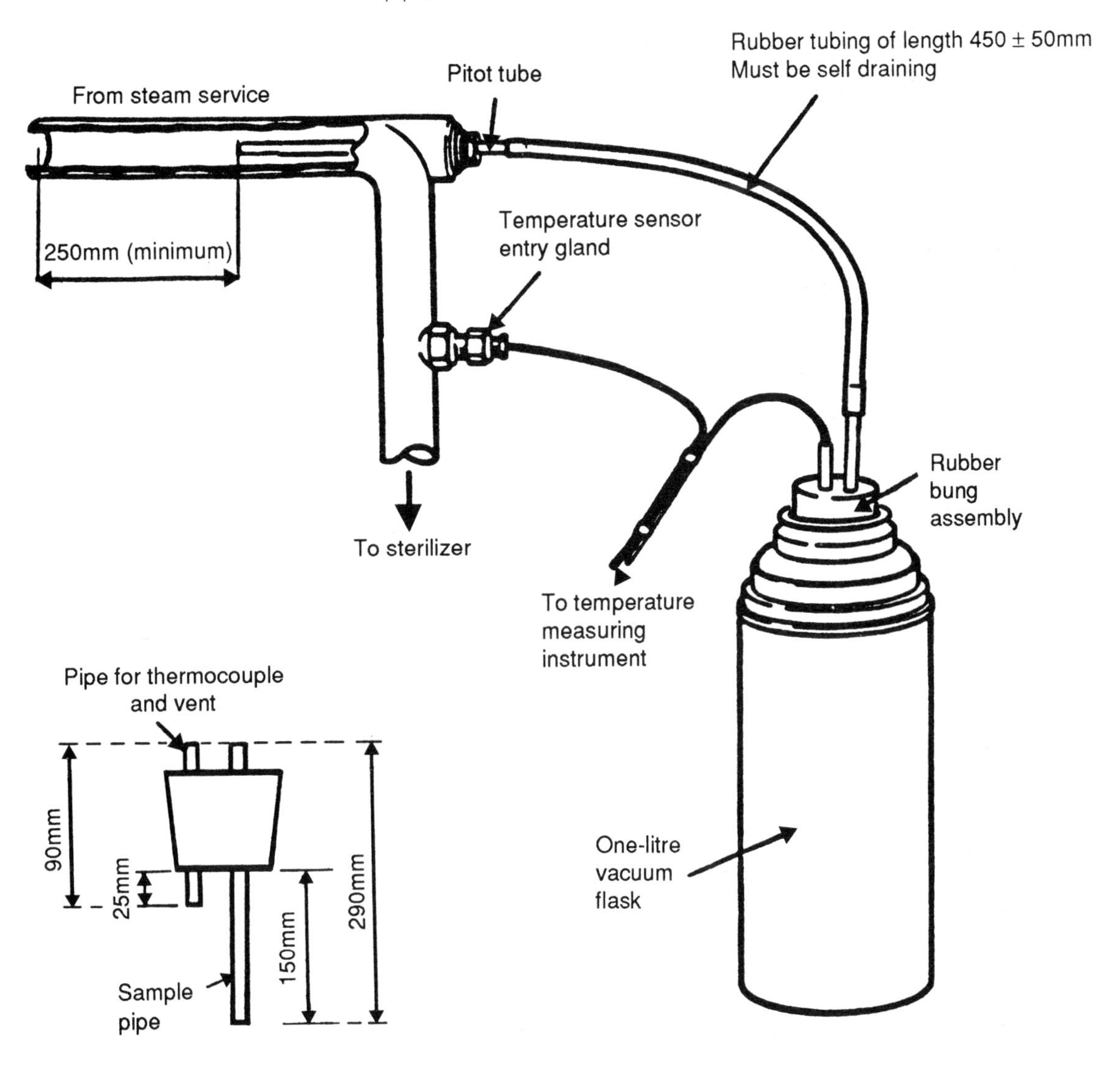

Figure 12 Apparatus for dryness test

9.35 Connect the rubber tube to the longer of the pipes in the stopper, place the stopper in the neck of the vacuum flask, weigh the whole assembly and note the mass (M_1).

9.36 Remove the stopper and tube assembly and pour 650 ± 50 ml of cold water (below 27°C) into the flask. Replace the stopper and tube assembly, weigh the flask and record the mass (M_2).

9.37 Support the flask close to the pitot, and ensure that the rubber tube and flask are protected from excess heat and draughts. Do not connect it to the pitot tube yet.

9.38 Introduce the second temperature sensor through the shorter of the two pipes in the stopper and into the water in the flask. Note the temperature of the water in the flask (T_0).

9.39 Ensure that the sterilizer chamber is empty except for the usual chamber furniture. Select and start the operating cycle.

9.40 When the steam supply to the chamber first opens, connect the rubber tube to the pitot discharge and wrap lagging around it. Arrange the rubber tube to permit condensate to drain freely into the flask. Note the temperature in the steam service pipe (T_s).

9.41 When the temperature of the water in the flask is approximately 80°C, disconnect the rubber tube from the pitot, agitate the flask so that the contents are thoroughly mixed, and note the temperature of the water (T_1).

9.42 Weigh the flask and stopper assembly and note the mass (M_3).

9.43 The initial mass of water in the flask is given by $M_w = M_2 - M_1$.

9.44 The mass of condensate collected is given by $M_c = M_3 - M_2$.

9.45 Calculate the dryness value of the steam from the following equation:

$$D = \frac{(T_1 - T_0)(4.18M_w + 0.24)}{LM_c} - \frac{4.18(T_s - T_1)}{L}$$

where:
T_0 = initial temperature of the water in the flask (°C);
T_1 = final temperature of the water and condensate in the flask (°C);
T_s = average temperature of the steam delivered to the sterilizer (°C);
M_w = initial mass of water in the flask (kg);
M_c = mass of condensate collected (kg);
L = latent heat of dry saturated steam at temperature T_s (kJ kg^{-1}).

9.46 A derivation of this equation, and a discussion of the assumptions implicit within it, can be found in Appendix 2.

9.47 The test should be considered satisfactory if the following requirements are met:

a. the dryness value is not less than 0.90 (if metal loads are to be processed, the dryness value should not be less than 0.95);

b. throughout the operating cycle, the temperature measured in the steam service pipe is within 3°C of that measured during the superheat test.

10.0 Sound pressure test

Introduction

10.1 British and European Standards require the manufacturer to carry out a sound power test as a type test for the sterilizer. This test, which measures the total radiated sound power from a sterilizer, must be performed in a suitably equipped test room and it is not necessary or practicable to repeat the test once a sterilizer has been installed.

10.2 Of more practical concern is the perceived level of noise in the immediate vicinity of the sterilizer. This quantity, the A-weighted sound pressure level, depends not only upon the sound power, but also upon the acoustic properties of the environment and other sources of noise. It must therefore be determined on site with the sterilizer installed and working normally. It follows that a failure of the sound pressure test need not imply that the sterilizer is faulty. It is possible that the machine is installed in a room with insufficient sound insulation. Information about sound-reducing measures may be found in Part 2 of this HTM.

10.3 The sound pressure test described in this chapter should be carried out according to the detailed instructions in BS4196: Part 6 (referred to in this chapter as BS4196). The additional information given here is by itself not sufficient to permit the test to be completed by personnel unfamiliar with the requirements of BS4196.

Test procedure

10.4 A precision sound-level meter is required as described in paragraph 6.51. The sound pressure levels are determined from a number of microphone positions. Where the measuring instrument has insufficient input channels, additional instruments or repeated operating cycles will be required.

10.5 The test determines the A-weighted sound pressure levels using a rectangular measurement surface. For the purpose of this test, the "reference surface" defined in BS4196 is to be drawn as follows:

a. for a single sterilizer, the reference surface is the smallest rectangular box that just encloses the sterilizer, with a width and depth measured from the outside of the vessel lagging, and a height measured from the floor to the top of the vessel lagging. The box does not include pipes and valves used to connect the sterilizer to its services;

b. for a group of sterilizers treated as a single source, the reference surface is the smallest rectangular box that just encloses the reference surfaces of the individual sterilizers.

10.6 Noise sources which contribute to the sound pressure level in the room in which the sterilizer is installed (including sources in adjacent rooms) should be operating during the test. In particular, all the building services in the area surrounding the room containing the sterilizer should be working normally, under their design conditions.

10.7 Sterilizers should be regarded as "large sound sources" as defined in BS4197. The measurement distance, *d*, should be 1.0 ± 0.1 m or half the distance from the sterilizer to an adjacent wall, whichever is less. It should not be less than 150 mm. Microphones should be placed in the following positions:

a. where a single sterilizer is the only major noise source in the room, place ten microphones as shown in Figure 13a. (If the sterilizer is recessed into a wall or partition, three of these microphones will be in the loading area and the remainder in the plantroom.) The microphone above the sterilizer may be omitted for safety reasons or if preliminary measurements show that its exclusion does not significantly affect the calculated value of the mean sound pressure level;

b. where several sterilizers are installed, they should be treated as a single large source and the reference surface drawn as described in paragraph 10.5b. Place ten microphones as shown in Figure 13b. If any dimension of the reference surface exceeds 5.0 m, intermediate microphone positions will be required as described in clause 7.4.3.2 of BS4196.

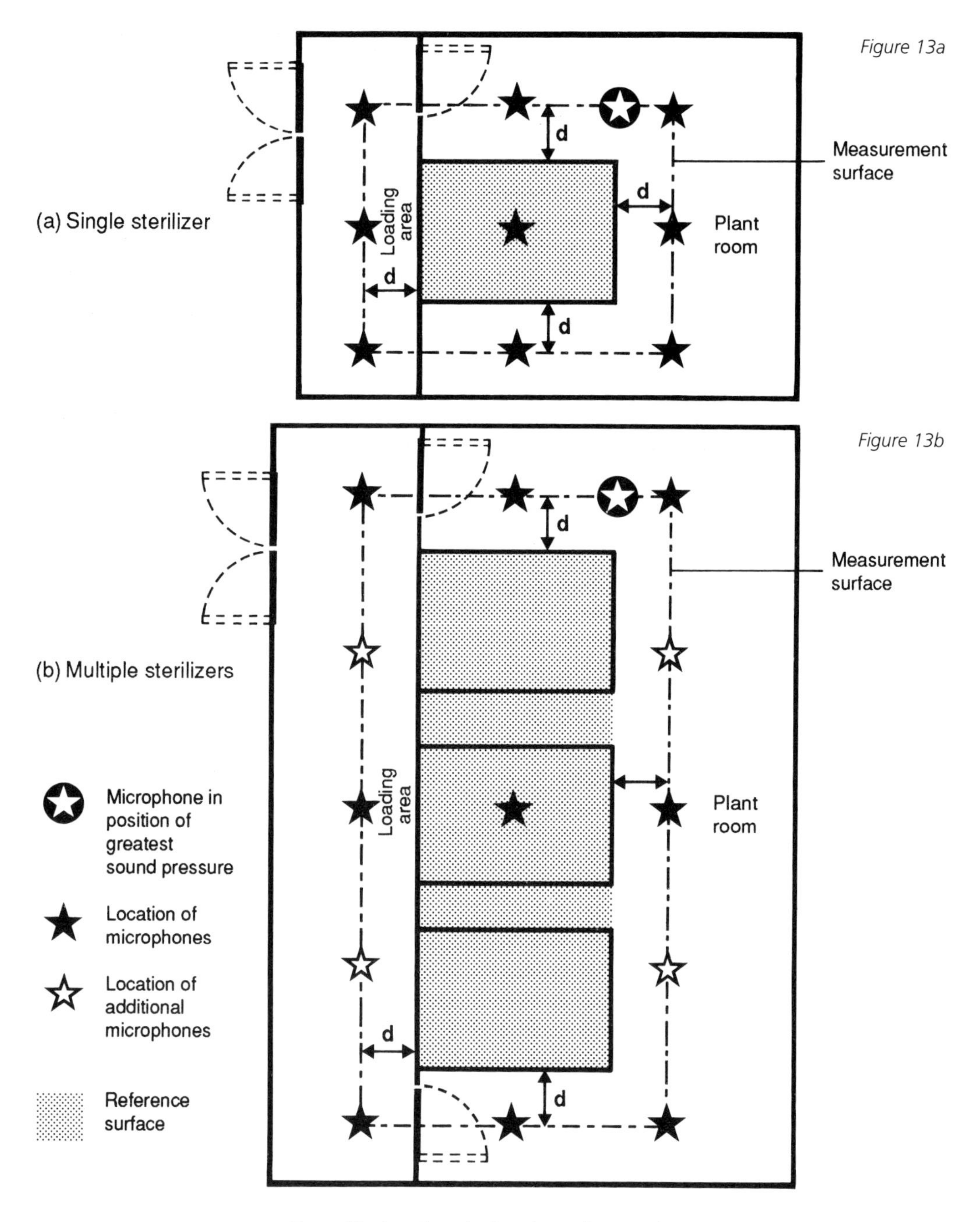

Figure 13 Location of microphones for sound pressure test

10.8 Load the sterilizer with a full load as described in the appropriate chapter of this HTM.

10.9 If there is a choice of operating cycle, select the cycle with the highest sterilization temperature. Ensure that the pressure and flow from the steam and water services are set to normal working levels. Start the operating cycle.

10.10 Integrate the sound pressure level throughout the operating cycle or, if the cycle exceeds 30 minutes, over a 30-minute period known to contain the loudest sounds.

10.11 Using the procedure described in clause 8.1 of BS4196, for both the plantroom and the loading area, determine the following:

a. the mean A-weighted surface sound pressure level;

b. the peak A-weighted surface sound pressure level.

10.12 The test should be considered satisfactory if the following requirements are met:

a. in the loading area, the mean A-weighted surface sound pressure level does not exceed:

   (i) 55 dBA for a sterilizer installed in an operating suite, pharmacy, treatment room or other noise-sensitive area;

   (ii) 70 dBA for a sterilizer installed in a sterile services department;

   (iii) 85 dBA for a sterilizer installed in an area that is not noise-sensitive;

b. in the plantroom, the mean A-weighted surface sound pressure level does not exceed 85 dBA;

c. in both the loading area and the plantroom, the peak A-weighted surface sound pressure level does not exceed the mean A-weighted surface sound pressure level by more than 15 dBA.

11.0 Chamber integrity tests

Introduction

11.1 These tests are designed to show that the sterilizer chamber does not leak either under vacuum or under pressure, and that the devices used to monitor leakage and the presence of air are functioning correctly.

Vacuum leak test

11.2 The vacuum leak test is applicable to any sterilizer which employs vacuum to remove air from the load, that is, porous load sterilizers, LTS disinfectors, LTSF sterilizers, EO sterilizers and some laboratory sterilizers.

11.3 Leakage of air into the chamber at a rate greater than that specified below (see paragraph 11.15) is unacceptable for three reasons:

a. the presence of air inhibits penetration of the load by the sterilant (steam or gas) and prevents sterilization;

b. air leaking into the chamber during the drying and air admission stages will not have passed through the bacteria-retentive filter, and therefore there is a risk of recontamination of the load;

c. the presence of air may cause an explosive hazard in EO sterilizers.

11.4 A vacuum leak test is required to establish that permissible limits are not exceeded.

11.5 The test is performed by measuring the change of vacuum in the chamber when all valves leading to it have been closed and the vacuum source isolated. If the test is conducted as part of a programme including thermometric tests, it will be necessary to repeat it with the temperature sensors and any test pressure gauge in place, and again when they have been removed, to ensure that there is no leakage through the ports. These tests are specified in the appropriate schedules in Chapters 4 and 5.

11.6 The test may either be part of the air removal stage or be performed at the end of the drying stage. It is designed to be carried out either automatically or semi-automatically, and in either case selected by a switch or data entry point located on the front fascia. It should be performed with an empty chamber.

11.7 If the sterilizer is not fitted with a vacuum leak test instrument, connect a 0–160 mbar absolute pressure gauge (Table 6) to the chamber.

11.8 For the test to be accurate, the chamber temperature should be stable. For example, in a closed vessel at 40 mbar absolute, the pressure changes by approximately 1 mbar for each 10°C change in temperature over the range 20–140°C. At 70 mbar the change is approximately 2 mbar. The test could be compromised if the temperature changes by more than 10°C during the period in which the chamber pressure is monitored. Stabilise the temperature of the chamber by one of the following methods:

a. if the vessel incorporates a heated jacket, carry out an operating cycle with the chamber empty;

b. if there is no heated jacket, ensure that the temperature of the chamber is no greater than 20°C from ambient.

11.9 When the temperature has stabilised, start the vacuum leak test cycle. For automatic systems the following steps are performed automatically, and the vacuum leak rate is displayed as a pressure rise in mbar min^{-1}. For semi-automatic systems, the pressures should be read and noted by the operator.

11.10 When the pressure in the chamber drops below 50 mbar absolute (or the maximum vacuum attained in an EO cycle), close all the valves connected to the chamber and stop the vacuum pump. Note the time and the absolute pressure (P_1).

11.11 Wait for 5 minutes (± 10 s), and then note the pressure again (P_2).

11.12 Wait for a further 10 minutes (± 10 s), and then note the pressure for a third time (P_3).

11.13 Restore the operating cycle, and allow it to proceed normally.

11.14 Calculate the vacuum leak rate for the 10-minute period from:

Vacuum leak rate = $(P_3 - P_2)/10$ mbar min^{-1}

11.15 For chambers with a capacity of 250–600 l, the test should be considered satisfactory if the following requirements are met:

a. the absolute pressure (P_2) at the start of the 10-minute period is:

(i) less than 70 mbar for porous load sterilizers, LTS disinfectors, LTSF sterilizers and laboratory sterilizers;

(ii) as specified by the manufacturer for EO sterilizers;

b. the vacuum leak rate does not exceed:

(i) 1.3 mbar min^{-1} for porous load sterilizers and laboratory sterilizers;

(ii) 0.5 mbar min^{-1} for LTS disinfectors and LTSF sterilizers;

(iii) 1.0 mbar min^{-1} for EO sterilizers.

11.16 For chambers outside the range 250–600 l, the test should be considered satisfactory if the pressure P_2 and the vacuum leak rate are as specified by the manufacturer.

11.17 Considerable care must be applied in the interpretation of the results of leak tests. On a typical test on a porous load sterilizer the pressure may rise by 20 mbar or more ($P_2 - P_1$) in the first 5 minutes of the test due to the evaporation of moisture remaining in the chamber and connecting pipework. Such a result does not necessarily indicate a leak.

11.18 A machine which fails to meet the requirements of this test should not be used until the fault has been rectified and the test satisfactorily completed.

Vacuum leak monitor test

11.19 For LTS disinfectors, and LTSF and EO sterilizers, the air removal stage is followed by an automatic check on the leakage of air into the chamber. The vacuum leak monitor test ensures that when the monitoring device is challenged with a specified leak rate the operating cycle is aborted and a fault is indicated.

11.20 Connect an air flow metering device (see paragraph 6.52) to the chamber.

11.21 Follow the procedure for the vacuum leak test, adjusting the metering device to cause a leak rate over the 10-minute test period of:

a. 5.0 ± 0.2 mbar min^{-1} for LTS disinfectors and LTSF sterilizers;

b. 3.0 ± 0.2 mbar min^{-1} for EO sterilizers.

11.22 For LTS disinfectors and LTSF sterilizers, place a standard test pack (see paragraph 7.27) in the chamber. For EO sterilizers, leave the chamber empty. Start the operating cycle.

11.23 The test should be considered satisfactory if the operating cycle is aborted after the air removal stage and a fault is indicated at the end of the cycle.

Pressure leak test

11.24 The pressure leak test is applicable to sterilizers which use EO or EO gas mixtures to sterilize products in chambers pressurised above atmospheric pressure.

11.25 Leakage of EO from the chamber at a rate greater than that specified below (see paragraph 11.35) is unacceptable because the gas is toxic and flammable. The maximum exposure limits are listed in Table 1. A pressure leak test is required to establish that leakage from the sterilizer will not cause these limits to be exceeded.

11.26 The test is performed by measuring the change of pressure in the chamber when all valves leading to it have been closed and the pressurising source has been isolated. If the test is conducted as part of a programme which includes thermometric tests, it will be necessary to repeat it with the temperature sensors and any test pressure gauge in place, and again when they have been removed, to ensure that there is no leakage through the ports. These tests are specified in the appropriate schedules in Chapters 4 and 5.

11.27 The test is performed using an inert gas as described in paragraph 1.29 and the measurements taken during the gas exposure stage. The test is designed to be carried out either automatically or semi-automatically, and in either case is selected by a switch or data entry point located on the front fascia. It should be performed with an empty chamber, immediately following a vacuum leak test.

11.28 If the sterilizer is not fitted with a pressure leak test instrument, connect a test gauge to the chamber. This should have a accuracy of 1% or better over a range of ± 10% of the gas exposure pressure.

11.29 Start the pressure leak test cycle. This is similar to a normal operating cycle except that an inert gas is used instead of EO. For automatic systems the following steps are performed automatically and the pressure leak rate is displayed as a pressure fall in mbar/min. For semi-automatic systems, the pressures are noted by the operator.

11.30 When the working pressure is attained, the gas will continue to be injected intermittently for a further 5 minutes to allow the pressure and temperature in the chamber to stabilise.

11.31 Close the valves connected to the chamber, and stop the pressure source. Observe and note the time and the pressure (P_1).

11.32 Wait for 60 ± 1 minutes and then observe and note the pressure again (P_2).

11.33 Restore the operating cycle, and allow it to proceed normally.

11.34 Calculate the pressure leak rate for the 60-minute period from:

Pressure leak rate = $(P_1 - P_2)/60$ mbar min^{-1}.

11.35 The test should be considered satisfactory if the following requirements are met:

a. for chambers with a capacity of 250–600 l, the pressure leak rate does not exceed 1.0 mbar min^{-1};

b. for chambers outside the range 250–600 l, the pressure leak rate is as specified by the manufacturer.

11.36 A machine which fails to meet the requirements of this test should not be used until the fault has been rectified.

Air detector tests

11.37 An air detector is fitted to certain sterilizers which employ vacuum as a means of removing air from the load before sterilization. It is currently required for porous load sterilizers and may also be fitted to LTS disinfectors, LTSF sterilizers and some laboratory sterilizers. It is used to determine whether any air or non-condensable gas present in the chamber is sufficient to impair the sterilizing process. The air detector should cause a fault to be indicated if the amount of air or gas in the chamber at the start of the plateau period is sufficient to depress the temperature in the centre of the load more than 2°C below the temperature in the active chamber discharge.

11.38 A correctly adjusted air detector will contribute to product security but should not be regarded as an alternative to effective maintenance.

11.39 The procedure for setting an air detector is lengthy and complex if prior information is not available. The manufacturer will have established the correct settings for the air detector and should supply the following information:

a. the setting of the sensitivity of the air detector;

b. the level of the signal from the air detector (the "trigger point"), which will trigger the automatic controller to abort the cycle and indicate a fault;

c. the vacuum leak rate that will cause this level to be exceeded.

11.40 The three air detector tests are designed to demonstrate compliance with the manufacturer's specifications. Several operating cycles will be required to complete the tests satisfactorily.

11.41 The three tests – for small load, full load and function – should be performed in sequence after it has been established that the vacuum leak rate of the sterilizer is acceptable.

11.42 Before starting the tests, connect an air-flow metering device (see paragraph 6.52) to the chamber by means of the valved port provided by the sterilizer manufacturer. It will normally be necessary to conduct a sequence of vacuum leak tests to establish the relationship between the setting on the metering device and the induced vacuum leak rate. The relationship should be recorded in the plant history file for each sterilizer.

11.43 If the sterilizer is not fitted with a leak test instrument, connect a 0–160 mbar absolute pressure test gauge (Table 6) to the chamber.

11.44 The two air detector performance tests require temperatures to be recorded by independent measuring equipment as described in Chapter 6.

Performance test for a small load

11.45 This test is designed to determine the setting for the air detector so that, with a small load, it will respond to a leak rate sufficient to depress the temperature in the test pack by no more than 2°C.

11.46 The procedure for the small-load test is set out in the flow chart in Figure 14. If the air detector is correctly set, the test should proceed rapidly down the left-hand branch and be complete in two cycles.

11.47 Select the operating cycle with the highest sterilization temperature and standard drying time.

11.48 Place a standard test pack (see paragraph 7.27) in the chamber, with the bottom of the pack supported 100–200 mm above the centre of the chamber base, and two temperature sensors placed in the following positions:

a. one in an active chamber discharge (see paragraph 6.26);

b. one at the approximate centre of the test pack (the wire from the sensor should be carefully arranged to prevent steam tracking along it).

11.49 A fresh test pack is required for each cycle. In practice, three test packs will be enough, provided that two are unfolded and left to air while the other is in the chamber.

11.50 At the start of the test ensure that the air detector sensitivity is set to the value recommended by the manufacturer. The detector can be disabled by adjusting the automatic controller so that it will not recognise a fault. This may be done by setting the trigger point, in accordance with the manufacturer's instructions, to a level that will not be attained during normal operation (see paragraph 11.39(b)).

11.51 During the air removal stage, admit air into the chamber by means of the metering device. From the measured temperatures, determine the temperature depression at the start of the plateau period:

Depression, $\Delta T = T_c - T_p$

where:
T_c = temperature measured in the active chamber discharge;
T_p = temperature measured in the centre of the test pack.

11.52 When the small-load test is complete, proceed immediately to the full-load test.

Performance test for a full load

11.53 This test is designed to show that an air detector set to respond correctly during the small-load test will also respond correctly with a full load. It is normally carried out immediately after a satisfactory completion of a small-load test.

11.54 The procedure for the full-load test is set out in the flow chart in Figure 15. If the air detector has been correctly set, the test should proceed rapidly down the left-hand branch and be complete in two cycles.

11.55 Select the operating cycle used for the small-load test.

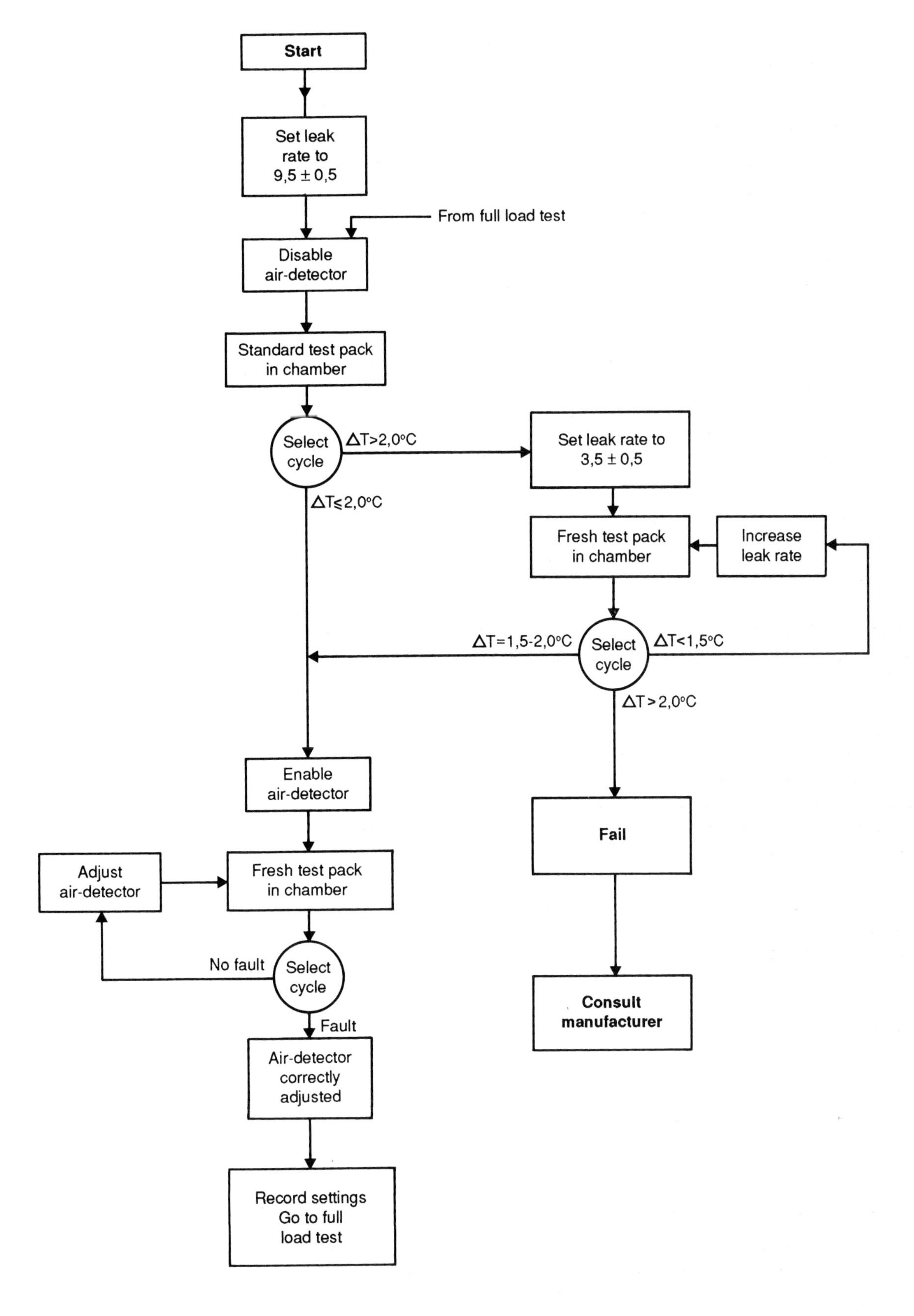

Leak rates in millibars/minute
Temperatures, ΔT, in °C

Figure 14 Procedure for air detector small-load test

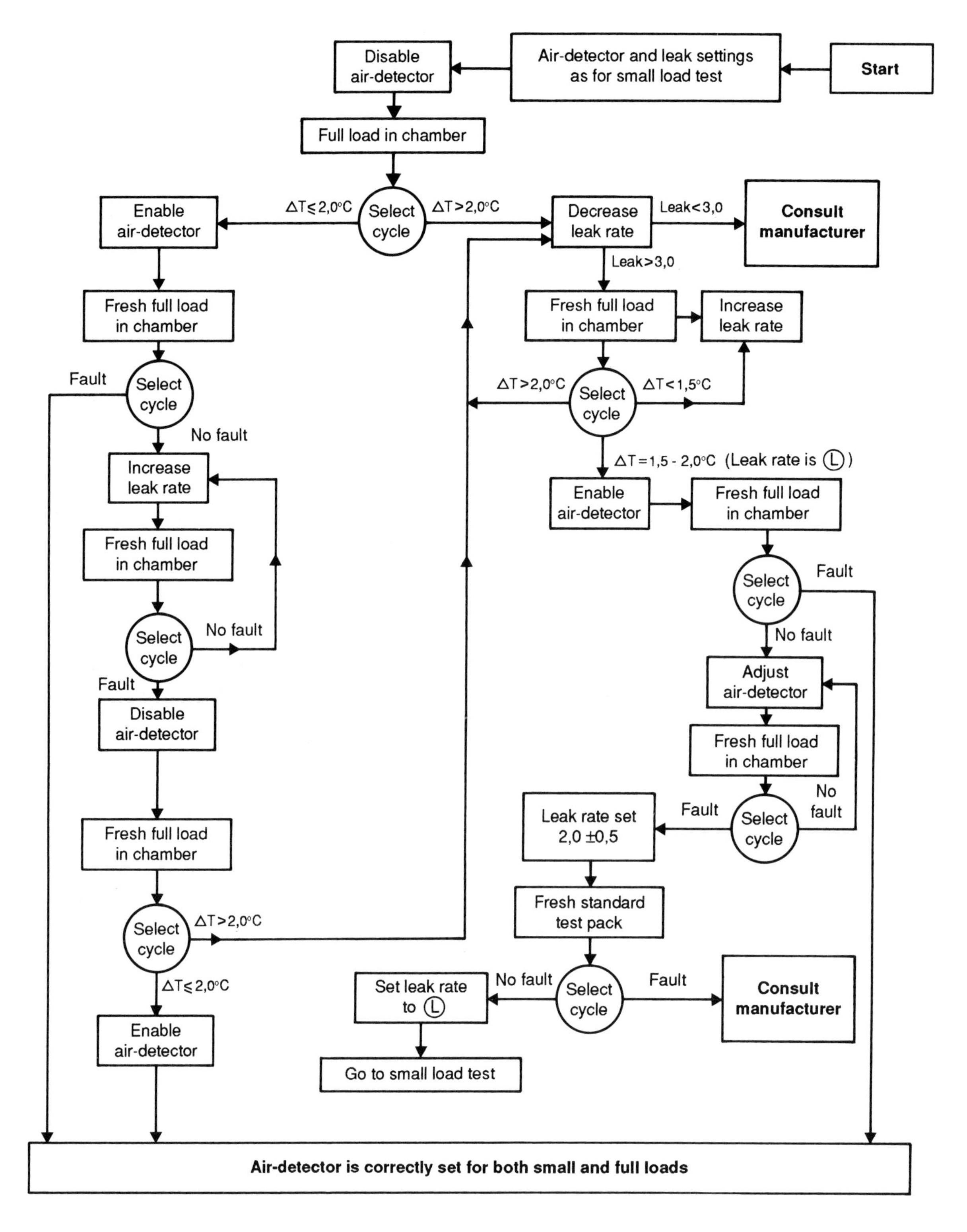

Figure 15 Procedure for air detector full load test

11.56 The load is a standard test pack placed in the chamber in a position identified by the manufacturer as the most difficult to sterilize, with the remaining usable chamber space filled with a full load appropriate to the type of sterilizer under test (see the procedure for the relevant thermometric test for a full load). Place temperature sensors as for the small-load test.

11.57 A fresh load is required for each cycle. In practice, three loads will be enough provided that two are unfolded and left to air while the other is in the chamber.

11.58 At the start of the test ensure that the air detector sensitivity and leak rate settings are identical to those established in the small-load test.

11.59 If, during the test, it becomes necessary to readjust the air detector, the procedure requires the small-load test to be repeated from the point indicated in Figure 13.

Function test

11.60 This test is designed to confirm that the air detector is functioning correctly during a normal operating cycle.

11.61 Set the air-flow metering device to the setting established during the small-load test.

11.62 Place a standard test pack in the chamber, with the bottom of the pack supported 100–200 mm above the centre of the chamber base.

11.63 Select and start the operating cycle.

11.64 The test should be considered satisfactory if the operating cycle is aborted and a fault is indicated. If the cycle is not aborted, then the advice of the manufacturer should be sought.

11.65 When the air detector tests are complete, the settings of the air detector sensitivity, the automatic controller trigger point, and the air-flow metering device and induced vacuum leak rate should be noted in the test report.

12.0 Automatic control test

Introduction

12.1 The automatic control test is designed to show that the operating cycle functions correctly as evidenced by the values of the cycle variables indicated and recorded by the instruments fitted to the sterilizer. It is carried out once a week on most sterilizers, and is the main test for ensuring that the sterilizer continues to function correctly.

12.2 During the commissioning, yearly and quarterly test programmes the temperature and pressure sensors for subsequent thermometric tests will be connected to the chamber during this test. If one sensor is placed in the active chamber discharge (see paragraph 6.26) the calibration of the sterilizer instruments may conveniently be checked during the holding time of the automatic control test.

Test procedure

12.3 For porous load sterilizers, LTS disinfectors and laboratory sterilizers (fabrics cycle), place a standard test pack (see paragraph 7.27) in the chamber, with the bottom of the pack supported 100–200 mm above the centre of the chamber base.

12.4 For sterilizers for unwrapped instruments and utensils, leave the chamber empty except for the usual chamber furniture.

12.5 For fluid, dry-heat, LTSF, EO and laboratory sterilizers:

a. for installation and commissioning tests, leave the chamber empty except for the usual chamber furniture;

b. for periodic tests, load the chamber with a production load of a type for which a record has been established during performance qualification. If the test proves satisfactory, the sterilized load may be released for normal use.

12.6 Sterilizers designed for fluid loads (fluid sterilizers, dry-heat sterilizers and certain laboratory sterilizers) are equipped with one or two probes to record the temperature of the load. If a production load is being processed, insert the probes into the load in the positions they would normally occupy. Otherwise stow the probes on the bracket provided in the chamber. Do not insert probes into discard material to be processed in laboratory make-safe cycles.

12.7 If an LTSF or EO sterilizer is being tested with an empty chamber, ensure that the sterilant is replaced with an inert substitute (see paragraph 1.29).

12.8 Select the sterilization temperature for the operating cycle to be tested. As a rule, this should be the highest temperature compatible with the load. If a production load is being used, select the temperature at which it would normally be sterilized. Start the cycle.

12.9 Ensure that a batch process record is made by the recording instrument fitted to the sterilizer. If the sterilizer does not have a recorder (such as some machines for unwrapped instruments and utensils), observe and note the elapsed time, indicated chamber temperatures and pressures at all significant points of the operating cycle, for example the beginning and end of each stage or sub-stage, and the maximum values during the holding time.

12.10 At the approximate mid-point of the plateau period, note the elapsed time and indicated chamber temperature and pressure.

12.11 For fluid loads, during the cooling stage wait for the temperature in the containers to fall to 95°C (plastic containers) or 85°C (glass). Wearing protective visor and gloves, attempt to open the door.

12.12 For fluid loads, as soon as the cycle is complete, but before opening the door, observe and note the recorded temperature in the containers.

12.13 The test should be considered satisfactory if the following requirements are met:

a. a visual display of "cycle complete" is indicated;

b. during the whole of the cycle the values of the cycle variables as shown on the batch process record are either within the limits established by the manufacturer as giving satisfactory results, or, for production loads, within the permitted tolerances marked on a master process record subsequently established during performance qualification;

c. during the plateau period determined from the recorded chamber temperature:

   (i) the indicated and recorded chamber temperatures are within the appropriate sterilization temperature band specified in Table 8;

   (ii) the difference between the indicated and recorded chamber temperature does not exceed 2°C;

   (iii) the difference between the indicated and recorded chamber pressure does not exceed 0.1 bar;

d. the holding time determined from any load temperature probes is not less than that specified in Table 8;

e. during the holding time, any temperatures recorded in the load are within the appropriate sterilization temperature band specified in Table 8;

f. the door cannot be opened until the cycle is complete;

g. for fluid loads, at the end of the cycle the temperature recorded in the containers is not greater than 90°C (plastic) or 80°C (glass);

h. the person conducting the test does not observe any mechanical or other anomaly.

13.0 Porous load sterilizers

Introduction

13.1 This chapter contains detailed procedures for tests specific to sterilizers designed to process porous loads. Schedules prescribing which tests are to be carried out and when are set out in Chapter 4 (for validation tests) and Chapter 5 (for periodic tests).

13.2 Unless specified otherwise, all the tests should be performed at each of the sterilization temperatures available on the sterilizer.

Chamber wall temperature test

13.3 This test is designed to show that temperature variations across the chamber walls do not exceed 2°C at the sterilization temperature. Temperatures and pressures should be recorded by independent measuring equipment as described in Chapter 6. The test is performed with an empty chamber.

13.4 Place 12 temperature sensors in the following positions:

a. one in an active chamber discharge (see paragraph 6.26);

b. five on each of the two chamber side walls (one at the approximate centre and four adjacent to the corner positions of the usable chamber space);

c. one on the plane of the usable chamber space (not on the wall), at a point nearest to the steam inlet port.

13.5 If a jacket is fitted, ensure that it is heated. Select and start the operating cycle.

13.6 The test should be considered satisfactory if, at the start of the plateau period, the measured temperatures are within 2°C of each other.

Thermometric test for a small load

13.7 This test is used to demonstrate that after the air removal stage of the operating cycle, sterilizing conditions are obtained within the chamber and standard test pack. The more air there is to remove, the more exacting will be the test; that is why the pack is used by itself in an otherwise empty chamber.

13.8 Temperatures and pressures should be recorded by independent measuring equipment as described in Chapter 6.

13.9 Place a standard test pack (see paragraph 7.27) in the chamber with the bottom of the pack supported 100–200 mm above the centre of the chamber base.

13.10 Place three temperature sensors in the following positions:

a. one in an active chamber discharge (see paragraph 6.26);

b. one at the approximate centre of the test pack (the wire from the sensor should be carefully arranged to prevent steam tracking along it);

c. one placed in the free space 50 ± 5 mm above the approximate centre of the upper surface of the test pack.

13.11 Connect a pressure recorder (or test gauge) to the chamber.

13.12 Start the operating cycle, with standard drying time, and take readings as described for the automatic control test (see paragraph 12.9).

13.13 If a test gauge is being used, measure the chamber pressure at the approximate mid-point of the holding time.

13.14 The test should be considered satisfactory if the following requirements are met:

a. the requirements of the automatic control test (see paragraph 12.13) are met;

b. during the plateau period the temperature measured above the test pack does not exceed the temperature measured in the active chamber discharge by more than 5°C for the first 60 s and 2°C for the remaining period;

c. the equilibration time determined from the measured temperatures does not exceed 15 seconds for chambers up to 800 l and 30 seconds for larger chambers;

d. the holding time determined from the measured temperatures is not less than that specified in Table 8;

e. during the holding time the temperatures measured in the active chamber discharge and in the centre of the test pack:
   (i) are within the appropriate sterilization temperature band specified in Table 8;
   (ii) do not fluctuate by more than ± 1°C;
   (iii) do not differ from one another by more than 2°C;

f. during the holding time:
   (i) the indicated and recorded chamber temperatures are within 1°C of the temperature measured in the active chamber discharge;
   (ii) the indicated and recorded chamber pressures are within 0.05 bar of the measured pressure;

g. for sterilizers using vacuum as the sole method of drying:
   (i) the duration of the drying stage is not less than 3 minutes;
   (ii) the chamber pressure at the end of the stage does not exceed 40 mbar absolute;

h. at the end of the cycle the sheets are sensibly dry.

Thermometric test for a full load

13.15 The full-load test is designed to demonstrate that, at the levels at which cycle variables are set, rapid and even penetration of steam into the centre of a load occurs, and the sterilizing condition is achieved in a test load of specified maximum mass and of sufficient size to fill the usable chamber space.

13.16 Temperatures and pressures should be recorded by independent measuring equipment as described in Chapter 6.

13.17 The load is made up of a standard test pack (see paragraph 7.27) and additional folded sheets designed to represent the maximum mass of textiles which may be processed in the sterilizer. Each sheet should contain at least 50% m/m of cotton fibre and have a surface density of approximately 200 g m^{-2}. They should be washed and aired as for the standard test pack (see paragraphs 7.30–31). After airing, the sheets should be folded to approximately 25 cm × 50 cm and laid one on top of the other to form stacks of mass 7.5 ± 0.5 kg.

13.18 Place the standard test pack within the chamber in a position identified by the manufacturer as the most difficult to sterilize. This will normally be in the approximate centre of the chamber.

13.19 Place three temperature sensors in the following positions:

a. one in an active chamber discharge (see paragraph 6.26);

b. one at the approximate centre of the test pack (the wire from the sensor should be carefully arranged to prevent steam tracking along it);

c. one below the approximate centre of the top sheet of the test pack.

13.20 Load the rest of the usable chamber space with stacks of sheets. (The mass of fabric in the load should be equivalent to 7.5 ± 0.5 kg for a unit volume 300 mm × 300 mm × 600 mm.)

13.21 Connect a pressure recorder (or test gauge) to the chamber.

13.22 Start the operating cycle, with standard drying time, and take readings as described for the automatic control test (see paragraph 12.9).

13.23 If a test gauge is being used, measure the chamber pressure at the approximate mid-point of the holding time.

13.24 The test should be considered satisfactory if the following requirements are met:

a. the requirements of the automatic control test (see paragraph 12.13) are met;

b. the equilibration time determined from the measured temperatures does not exceed 15 s for chambers up to 800 l and 30 s for larger chambers;

c. the holding time determined from the measured temperatures is not less than that specified in Table 8;

d. during the holding time:

   (i) the measured temperatures are within the appropriate sterilization temperature band specified in Table 8;

   (ii) the measured temperatures do not fluctuate by more than ± 1°C;

   (iii) the measured temperatures do not differ from one another by more than 2°C;

   (iv) the indicated and recorded chamber temperatures are within 1°C of the temperature measured in the active chamber discharge;

   (v) the indicated and recorded chamber pressures are within 0.05 bar of the measured pressure;

e. the total cycle time is within the performance class stated by the manufacturer;

f. at the end of the cycle the sheets are sensibly dry.

Load dryness test

13.25 This test is used to demonstrate that the operating cycle, without extended drying, will not cause an increase in moisture in a standard test pack sufficient for there to be uncertainty about the dryness of loads routinely processed.

13.26 Three polythene bags, at least 35 cm × 25 cm and of polythene at least 250 µm thick, and a balance capable of weighing loads up to 2 kg with an accuracy of 0.1 g or better, are required.

13.27 Allow the sheets which will comprise the standard test pack to air as described in paragraph 7.31.

13.28 Mark three of the sheets and similarly mark each of the polythene bags so that each sheet is identified with a bag.

13.29 Weigh each of the polythene bags and note the mass (M_1).

13.30 Place each sheet in a polythene bag, weigh each bag with its enclosed sheet and note the mass (M_2).

13.31 Remove the sheets from the bags and assemble the standard test pack with one of the sheets in the centre of the pack and one in the second position from each end of the pack.

13.32 Place the test pack in the approximate centre of the sterilizer chamber and start the operating cycle within one minute. (Extended drying should not be used.)

13.33 Not more than one minute after the cycle has finished, remove the test pack from the chamber. Remove the three sheets from the test pack and put them quickly into their marked bags. Seal each bag by turning its open end over several times. This operation should be completed as quickly as possible to reduce evaporation of retained moisture and in any case within three minutes of the end of the cycle.

13.34 Weigh each bag with its enclosed sheet and note the mass (M_3).

13.35 Calculate the percentage gain in mass of each sheet from the formula:

$$\text{percentage gain in mass} = 100 \times \frac{(M_3 - M_2)}{(M_2 - M_1)}$$

13.36 The test should be considered satisfactory if the average gain in mass of each of the three bagged sheets is not more than 1%.

Hospital load dryness check

13.37 Process a production load which is known to present the greatest challenge to the operating cycle. Extended drying may be required.

13.38 The check should be considered satisfactory if a "cycle complete" indication is obtained and the load is sensibly dry.

Bowie-Dick test for steam penetration

13.39 Sterilization is achieved by the rapid and even penetration of steam into all parts of the load and the maintenance of these conditions for the specified holding time. To ensure this, it is essential to remove air from the chamber and load, and to provide a steam supply which contains a minimal volume of non-condensable gases. Any residual air and non-condensable gases will become concentrated as a bubble in the load and inhibit steam penetration.

13.40 The Bowie-Dick test shows whether or not steam penetration of the test pack is even and rapid, and thus by implication that air or other non-condensable gases are not present. It does not confirm that the sterilization conditions in the load have been achieved.

Principle of the test

13.41 The test, as originally conceived and described in earlier editions of HTM 10 (Bowie, Kelsey and Thomson, 1963), is based on the use of a chemical indicator in the form of an adhesive tape stuck to a piece of suitable paper to form a St Andrew's cross. This indicator paper is placed at the centre of a test pack of folded huckaback towels and then subjected to an operating cycle. The indicator tape shows a change of colour in response to a combination of time, temperature and moisture.

13.42 If no air is present in the chamber, steam will penetrate rapidly and completely, and the indicator will show a uniform colour change. If air is present, it will collect within the pack as a bubble. The indicator in the region of the bubble will be of a different colour than elsewhere on the paper, because of a lower temperature, lower moisture level or both.

13.43 The modern Bowie-Dick test uses a Class B chemical indicator conforming to EN 867: Part 3 (see paragraph 7.40) contained within a standard test pack (see paragraph 7.27). The indicator is distributed over an A4 paper sheet in the form of a geometric pattern.

13.44 When used in conjunction with a standard test pack, Class B indicators are designed to show a failure either if, at the start of the holding time, the temperature at the centre of the test pack is 2°C or more below the temperature in the active chamber discharge; or if the indicator is exposed to insufficient moisture. Both conditions are usually caused by the presence of air or other non-condensable gases (see paragraph 13.56). Because of the tolerances necessary in the manufacture of chemical indicators, users should be aware that in order to detect a temperature difference of 2°C the indicator may show signs of failure with a smaller temperature difference.

Test procedure

13.45 The Bowie-Dick test is normally preceded by a warm-up cycle. This cycle is necessary because the effectiveness of air removal may depend on all parts of the sterilizer being at working temperature. A satisfactory sterilizer may give a fail result if this is not done.

13.46 Remove the wrapping from a standard test pack and place the indicator paper in the sheet located nearest to the centre of the pack. Reassemble and secure the pack and replace the wrapping.

13.47 Place the test pack in the chamber with the bottom of the pack supported 100–200 mm above the centre of the chamber base.

13.48 Select the Bowie-Dick test cycle. Ensure that the holding time will not be longer than that specified in Table 10. If this time is exceeded, the indicator may change in such a way as to make it difficult to detect the variations that would indicate a fail condition. Start the operating cycle.

Sterilization temperature	Holding time	
	minimum	maximum
[°C]	[min]	[min]
134	3.3	3.5
126	10.8	11.0
121	16.8	17.0

Table 10 Holding times for the Bowie-Dick test cycle

13.49 During the holding time, note the reading on the cycle counter, the chamber temperature indicator and the chamber pressure indicator.

13.50 When the cycle is complete, remove the indicator paper from the test pack.

13.51 The test should be considered satisfactory if the following requirements are met:

a. there is a uniform change throughout the indicator;

b. the automatic controller indicates that a Bowie-Dick test cycle has just been completed.

13.52 It is important to compare the colour of the indicator at the corners of the paper with that at the centre so that any difference can be clearly seen. If there is any discernible difference the test should be recorded as failed, and the paper marked accordingly. A large area of unchanged indicator points to a gross failure.

13.53 The indicator paper should be marked with the result and kept for reference for at least three months. The chemical reaction continues during this time and the paper may be discarded when the indicator becomes unreadable. The associated batch process record should be kept for at least 11 years.

13.54 An unsatisfactory test result indicates that the machine should not be used until the fault has been rectified. It is important to realise that if a sterilizer fails to pass the Bowie-Dick test it cannot be made safe simply by increasing the holding time until a uniform colour change is produced. A failed sterilizer is in urgent need of skilled attention.

13.55 Several factors may inhibit steam penetration and cause the test to fail. Common causes of failure include the following:

a. an inefficient air removal stage;

b. an air leak during the air removal stage;

c. the presence of non-condensable gases in the steam supply.

13.56 A subsequent thermometric test for a small load (see paragraph 13.7) will assist in diagnosing the cause of failure:

a. if the test reveals a temperature depression at the centre of the test pack, the problem is likely to be inefficient air removal or an air leak into the chamber. Air remaining in the centre of the test pack is inhibiting the penetration of steam and the correct temperature is not being attained. The sterilizer should not be returned to service until it has been subjected to a vacuum leak test (see paragraph 11.2) and an air detector function test (see paragraph 11.60);

b. if the test fails to reveal a temperature depression, the problem is almost certainly air or other non-condensable gases in the steam supply. In this case the correct temperature is being attained but the steam is diluted, and insufficient moisture is present to change the indicator. The sterilizer should not be returned to service until the steam supply has been tested for the presence of non-condensable gases (see paragraph 9.4).

14.0 Fluid sterilizers

Introduction

14.1 This chapter contains detailed procedures for tests specific to sterilizers designed to process aqueous fluids in sealed containers. Schedules prescribing which tests are to be carried out and when are set out in Chapter 4 (for validation tests) and Chapter 5 (for periodic tests).

14.2 Unless specified otherwise, all the tests should be performed at each of the sterilization temperatures available on the sterilizer.

14.3 For the thermometric tests the containers should be filled with the nominal volume of water. The volumes of the fluid in each container should not differ from their mean by more than 5%. At the start of the cycle the temperature of the fluid in each container should be 20 ± 5°C.

Heat exchanger integrity test

14.4 This test is designed to check the integrity of the heat exchanger used to heat and cool the circulating coolant (air or water) in the sterilizer chamber. The circuit which is directly heated is called the primary circuit. Water in the primary circuit must be assumed to be non-sterile. The circuit which exposes coolant to the load is called the secondary circuit. In recent models of fluid sterilizers the secondary circuit is designed to operate at a higher pressure than the primary to prevent leakage of contaminated water into the chamber.

14.5 Where the heat exchanger is designed and constructed in a fail-safe fashion so that the secondary coolant cannot become contaminated under any circumstances, the test is required only for commissioning and yearly tests.

14.6 Attach a pressure recorder (or test gauge) to the primary circuit. The range should include the maximum pressure to which the circuit is to be pressurised.

14.7 Charge the primary circuit with water and pressurise it to either 1.5 times its maximum working pressure or twice the maximum pressure in the secondary circuit, whichever is less. This should be done in accordance with the manufacturer's instructions, and in some cases may require additional ports and valves to be fitted.

14.8 Close the inlet and outlet valves, and allow the pressure to stabilise over a period of 10 min. Observe and note the measured pressure. Wait for a further 10 min. Observe and note the pressure again.

14.9 The test should be considered satisfactory if the measured pressure has not fallen over the 10-min period.

Thermometric test for a full load

14.10 Temperatures and pressures should be recorded by independent measuring equipment as described in Chapter 6.

14.11 Load the chamber with one-litre bottles (nominal capacity), each filled with 1 l of water, at the minimum spacing recommended by the manufacturer. The bottles and chamber furniture should fill the usable chamber space. If the sterilizer is not designed to process one-litre bottles, the largest size recommended by the sterilizer manufacturer should be used.

14.12 Place 10 or 11 temperature sensors in the following positions:

a. one in an active chamber discharge (see paragraph 6.26);

b. one in each of the three bottles that are the slowest to attain the sterilization temperature;

c. one in each of the three bottles that are the fastest to attain the sterilization temperature;

d. one in each of the three bottles that are the slowest to cool to 90°C (plastic) or 80°C (glass);

e. one in the coolest part of the coolant spray system (if fitted).

14.13 Insert the load temperature probe into a bottle adjacent to the bottle identified as the slowest to attain the sterilization temperature. If a second probe is provided, insert it into a bottle adjacent to the bottle identified as the fastest to attain the sterilization temperature.

14.14 Connect a pressure recorder (or test gauge) to the chamber and, for sterilizers fitted with a spray pump, to the spray pump discharge. Where the heat exchanger secondary circuit is designed to operate at a higher pressure than the primary circuit, connect a third sensor to measure the differential pressure between the circuits.

14.15 Select and start the operating cycle and take readings as described for the automatic control test (see paragraph 12.9).

14.16 If a test gauge is being used, measure the chamber pressure at the approximate mid-point of the holding time.

14.17 As soon as the cycle is complete, note the measured temperature in the bottles before opening the door.

14.18 If required, collect a sample of coolant for a subsequent coolant quality test (see paragraph 14.32).

14.19 If the coolant is derived from a water or steam service, and is intended to come into contact with the load containers, the operating cycle must expose the coolant to sufficient heat to ensure that it is free of microbial contamination by the end of the holding time. This is checked by calculating an F_0 value (see Part 4 for a discussion of the use of F_0) that is equivalent to the time in minutes at a sterilization temperature of 121°C. If the test recorder is not capable of calculating F_0 (see paragraph 6.16), proceed as follows:

a. from the measured temperatures, identify the point during the heat-up time at which the coolant temperature first reaches 108°C. Note the temperature (T °C) at subsequent one-minute intervals until the end of the holding time;

b. for each measurement, calculate the incremental F_0 (ΔF_0) from the following equation:

$$\Delta F_0 = \log_{10}\left(\frac{T-121}{10}\right) \text{ minutes;}$$

c. the F_0 value is the sum of all ΔF_0.

14.20 The test should be considered satisfactory if the following requirements are met:

a. the requirements of the automatic control test (paragraph 12.13) are met;

b. the holding time is not less than that specified for the appropriate sterilization temperature band in Table 8;

c. during the holding time:

  (i) the measured temperatures are within the appropriate sterilization temperature band specified in Table 8;

  (ii) the measured temperatures are within 1°C of each other;

  (iii) the indicated and recorded chamber temperatures are within 1°C of the temperature measured in the active chamber discharge;

  (iv) the indicated and recorded chamber pressures are within 0.05 bar of the measured pressure;

  (v) the recorded chamber pressure is within 0.05 bar of saturated steam pressure or, if a partial pressure system is used, as specified by the manufacturer;

d. at the end of the cycle:

  (i) the temperature sensors have remained in position;

  (ii) the bottles containing sensors have not leaked, burst or broken;

  (iii) not more than one of the other bottles (or 1%, whichever is the greater) has burst or broken;

  (iv) the temperature measured in the bottles is not greater than 90°C (plastic) or 80°C (glass);

e. throughout the cycle:

  (i) the coolant spray pressure complies with the manufacturer's specifications;

  (ii) the pressure in the heat exchanger secondary circuit is greater than that in the primary circuit (if appropriate);

f. F_0 for the coolant is not less than 8 minutes;

g. the total cycle time is within the performance class stated by the manufacturer.

Thermometric test for a small load

14.21 Temperatures and pressures should be recorded by independent measuring equipment as described in Chapter 6.

14.22 Place 25 vials or ampoules of 5-ml nominal capacity, each containing 5 ml of water, in each of two wire baskets. Support one basket in the upper rear half of the usable chamber space and the other in the lower front half. Use the upper and lower shelves if provided. If the sterilizer is not designed to process vials or ampoules of this size, the smallest size and number of containers recommended by the sterilizer manufacturer should be used. Where the sterilizer is to be used to process one size of container only, the test load may be a single container of this size, filled with the nominal volume of water and supported in a position known to be the slowest to attain the sterilization temperature.

14.23 Place temperature sensors and load temperature probes as described for the full-load test.

14.24 Connect a pressure recorder (or test gauge) to the chamber and other pressure sensors as described for the full-load test.

14.25 Follow the procedure for the full-load test.

14.26 The test should be considered satisfactory if, except for paragraph 14.20 (g), the requirements of the full-load test (see paragraph 14.20) are met.

Simplified thermometric test for performance requalification

14.27 This test is not a substitute for a full PRQ test, but is used quarterly to check that the sterilization conditions continue to be met. Temperatures and pressures should be recorded by independent measuring equipment as described in Chapter 6.

14.28 Prepare a production load known to present the greatest challenge to the operating cycle and for which there is a PQ report. (This will normally be the reference load used in the yearly PRQ tests.)

14.29 Place three or four temperature sensors in the following positions:

a. one in an active chamber discharge (see paragraph 6.26);

b. one in a container that is the slowest to attain the sterilization temperature;

c. for chambers of capacity of 800 l and above, one in a container that is the fastest to attain the sterilization temperature;

d. one in a container that is the slowest to cool to 80°C (glass) or 90°C (plastic).

14.30 Place the load in the chamber as described in the PQ report. Select and start the operating cycle.

14.31 The test should be considered satisfactory if the requirements listed in the PQ report are met.

Coolant quality test

14.32 This test measures the concentration of particulates and dissolved solids in the coolant. It is carried out after a satisfactory operating cycle, normally at the end of a full-load, small-load or PQ test.

14.33 Rinse a one-litre bottle with purified water BP immediately before use and discard the rinsings.

14.34 Use the bottle to collect a test sample of cooling water from the coolant system immediately after an operating cycle but before the final discharge to waste.

14.35 Take a dish or beaker, made of silica or borosilicate glass, of capacity at least 150 ml. Dry the dish for 2 h in an oven at a temperature of 110 ± 2 °C. Put it in a desiccator and allow it to cool to ambient temperature. Weigh it to the nearest 0.1 mg and note the mass (M_1).

14.36 Ensuring that the test sample is well mixed, measure 100 ml of the test sample into the dish and evaporate it over a boiling-water bath until apparently dry.

14.37 Repeat with two further 100 ml of test sample transferred into the same dish.

14.38 Put the dish into the oven and heat at a temperature of 110 ± 2 °C for about 2 h. Put it in the desiccator and allow it to cool to ambient temperature. Weigh it to the nearest 0.1 mg and note the mass (M_2).

14.39 Repeat paragraph 14.38 until the difference between two consecutive weighings does not exceed 0.2 mg.

14.40 Calculate the concentration of residue in milligrams per litre of cooling water.

$$\text{Concentration of residue} = \frac{(M_2 - M_1)}{V} \text{ mg } l^{-1}$$

where:
M_1 = mass of dry dish (mg);
M_2 = final mass of dish and residue (mg);
V = volume of sample water evaporated (normally 300 ml).

14.41 The test should be considered satisfactory if the concentration of residue does not exceed 40 mg l^{-1}.

15.0 Sterilizers for unwrapped instruments and utensils

Introduction

15.1 This chapter contains detailed procedures for tests specific to sterilizers designed to process unwrapped solid instruments and utensils. Schedules, prescribing which tests are to be carried out and when, are set out in Chapter 4 (for validation tests) and Chapter 5 (for periodic tests). Except where stated otherwise, the tests in this chapter apply equally to fixed and transportable sterilizers.

15.2 Unless specified otherwise, all the tests should be performed at each of the sterilization temperatures available on the sterilizer.

Chamber overheat cut-out test

15.3 This test applies only to sterilizers where the steam is generated within the chamber. The test is done with an empty chamber and with insufficient water charge for a complete cycle. Temperatures should be recorded by independent measuring equipment as described in Chapter 6.

15.4 Attach a temperature sensor to the chamber wall in a position identified by the manufacturer as attaining the highest temperature.

15.5 Select the operating cycle with the highest sterilization temperature. (Only one cycle is normally provided.) Start the cycle.

15.6 The test should be considered satisfactory if the following requirements are met:

a. a boil-dry condition occurs before the end of the cycle;

b. the overheat cut-out operates, and the heaters are isolated from the electricity supply;

c. the chamber wall temperature does not exceed the temperature specified by the manufacturer.

Thermometric test for a small load

15.7 Temperatures and pressures should be recorded by independent measuring equipment as described in Chapter 6.

15.8 Place a pair of forceps (for example 5-inch artery forceps) in the approximate centre of the chamber.

15.9 Place three temperature sensors in the following positions:

a. one in an active chamber discharge (see paragraph 6.26);

b. one trapped between the jaws of the forceps;

c. where steam is supplied from outside the chamber, one in the upper third of the free chamber space;

d. where steam is generated within the chamber, one either in the reservoir or, if water is retained in the chamber, in the water.

15.10 Connect a pressure recorder (or test gauge) to the chamber.

15.11 Select and start the operating cycle.

15.12 The test should be considered satisfactory if the following requirements are met:

a. the requirements of the automatic control test (see paragraph 12.13) are met;

b. during the first minute of the plateau period the temperature measured in the chamber free space does not exceed the temperature measured in the active chamber discharge by more than 5°C;

c. after the first minute of the plateau period:

   (i) the temperature measured in the chamber free space does not exceed the temperature measured in the active chamber discharge by more than 2°C;

   (ii) the temperature measured in the jaws of the forceps is within 1°C of the temperature measured in the active chamber discharge;

d. the holding time determined from the measured temperatures is not less than that specified in Table 8;

e. during the holding time:

   (i) the measured temperatures are within the appropriate sterilization temperature band specified in Table 8;

   (iii) the indicated and recorded chamber temperatures are within 1°C of the temperature measured in the active chamber discharge;

   (v) the indicated and recorded chamber pressures are within 0.05 bar of the measured chamber pressure;

f. at the end of the cycle the temperature of any water left in the chamber or in the reservoir is less than the boiling point of water at local atmospheric pressure.

Thermometric test for a full load

15.13 Temperatures and pressures should be recorded by independent measuring equipment as described in Chapter 6.

15.14 Place a pair of forceps as for the small-load test in the approximate centre of the chamber, and add further instruments and utensils up to the maximum total mass which the sterilizer is designed to process.

15.15 Place four temperature sensors in the following positions:

a. one in an active chamber discharge (see paragraph 6.26);

b. one trapped between the jaws of the forceps;

c. where steam is supplied from outside the chamber, one in the free space between the load items;

d. where steam is generated within the chamber, one either in the reservoir or, if water is retained in the chamber, in the water.

15.16 Connect a pressure recorder (or test gauge) to the chamber.

15.17 Select and start the operating cycle.

15.18 The test should be considered satisfactory if the requirements for the small-load test are met, and the total cycle time is within the performance class stated by the manufacturer.

16.0 Dry-heat sterilizers

Introduction

16.1 This chapter contains detailed procedures for tests specific to dry-heat sterilizers. Schedules, prescribing which tests are to be carried out and when, are set out in Chapter 4 (for validation tests) and Chapter 5 (for periodic tests).

16.2 For these tests it is essential that load items are packaged and positioned in a manner which will permit the circulation of air to all parts of the chamber and pack surfaces.

16.3 Unless specified otherwise, all the tests should be performed at each of the sterilization temperatures available on the sterilizer.

Automatic control test

16.4 Follow the general procedure for the automatic control test given in Chapter 12 with the following amendments.

16.5 Where the chamber is pressurised during the cooling stage, note the differential pressure across the air filter after the start of the cooling stage and shortly before the end.

16.6 As soon as the cycle is complete, and before opening the door, note any recorded temperatures in the load containers.

16.7 The test should be considered satisfactory if the following requirements are met:

a. a visual indication of "cycle complete" is obtained;

b. during the whole of the cycle the values of the cycle variables as shown on the batch process record are either within the limits established by the manufacturer as giving satisfactory results, or within the permitted tolerances marked on a master process record subsequently established during performance qualification;

c. during the plateau period determined from the recorded chamber temperature:

   (i) the indicated and recorded chamber temperatures are within the appropriate sterilization temperature band specified in Table 8;

   (ii) the difference between the indicated and recorded chamber temperature does not exceed 5°C;

   (iii) the recorded chamber temperature does not drift by more than 2°C;

d. the holding time determined from any load temperature probes is not less than that specified in Table 8;

e. during the holding time, the recorded temperature in the load containers is within 5°C of the recorded chamber temperature;

f. during the cooling stage, the differential pressure indicated across the air filter is in the range specified by the manufacturer;

g. the door cannot be opened until the cycle is complete;

h. at the end of the cycle the temperature recorded in any load containers is not greater than 90°C;

j. the person conducting the test does not observe any mechanical or other anomaly.

Chamber overheat cut-out test

16.8 This test is designed to show that the thermal cut-out will prevent the temperature in the chamber from exceeding 200°C. The test should be done with an empty chamber. Temperatures should be recorded by independent measuring equipment as described in Chapter 6.

16.9 Place a temperature sensor in the hottest part of the chamber free space.

16.10 Inactivate the chamber temperature control to allow the temperature to rise. This should be done in accordance with the manufacturer's instructions.

16.11 Select and start the operating cycle.

16.12 The test should be considered satisfactory if the measured chamber temperature does not exceed 200°C during the cycle.

Air filter integrity test

16.13 This test is designed to show whether the high-efficiency particulate filter fitted to a dry-heat sterilizer is intact and working correctly. It is based on the test given in Appendix C of BS5295: Part 1.

16.14 A test aerosol generator and a photometer are required as described in Chapter 6.

16.15 The sterilizer should be at room temperature with the chamber door open. In accordance with the manufacturer's instructions, arrange for the chamber pressurising fan to be drawing air through the filter at its normal rate.

16.16 Set up the aerosol generator outside the chamber so that a uniform concentration of particles is dispersed across the intake of the air filter and its sealing frame. Ensure that this concentration is maintained throughout the test.

16.17 Using the photometer, measure the concentration of particles as close as possible to the intake of the filter and ideally not more than 150 mm from the filter face. Adjust the photometer (and the aerosol generator if necessary) to give a stable reading of 100%.

16.18 Inside the chamber, use the photometer to scan all of the downstream face of the filter including the sealing device. Hold the sampling probe approximately 25 mm away from the area being tested, and pass it over the entire area in slightly overlapping strokes at a traverse rate of no more than 50 mm s^{-1}. Make separate passes around the entire periphery of the filter, along the bond between the filter pack and the frame, and around the seal between the filter and retaining device.

16.19 Note the location of any steady, repeatable reading of the photometer.

16.20 The test should be considered satisfactory if any steady and repeatable reading does not exceed 0.001%.

16.21 A filter that fails the test should be replaced. It is not possible to repair the high-efficiency filters installed in dry-heat sterilizers.

Thermometric test for performance qualification

16.22 Temperatures should be recorded by independent measuring equipment.

16.23 Follow the procedure for the thermometric test for performance qualification given in Chapter 8 (see paragraph 8.13), but instead of placing a temperature sensor in an active chamber discharge place two sensors as follows:

a. one (sensor A) in thermal contact with the sensor connected to the sterilizer temperature recorder;

b. one (sensor B) in thermal contact with the sensor connected to the sterilizer temperature indicator.

16.24 Where the chamber is pressurised during the cooling stage, connect a pressure recorder to measure the differential pressure across the air filter. Measure the differential pressure during the cooling stage.

16.25 The test should be considered satisfactory if the following requirements are met:

a. the requirements of the automatic control test (see paragraph 16.7) are met;

b. the holding time, as determined from the measured temperatures, is not less than that specified in Table 8;

c. during the holding time:

   (i) the measured temperatures are within the appropriate sterilization temperature band specified in Table 8;

   (ii) the indicated chamber temperature is within 1°C of the temperature measured by sensor B;

   (iii) the recorded chamber temperature is within 1°C of the temperature measured by sensor A;

   (iv) the temperatures measured by each sensor in the load and by sensor B are within 5°C of the temperature measured by sensor A;

   (v) the temperature measured by sensor A does not drift more than 2°C;

d. during the cooling stage, the differential pressure measured across the air filter is in the range specified by the manufacturer;

e. at the end of the cycle:

   (i) the temperature sensors have remained in position;

   (ii) the items containing sensors are intact;

   (iii) the temperature measured in any item is not greater than 90°C.

Simplified thermometric test for performance requalification

16.26 This test is not a substitute for a full PRQ test, but is used quarterly to check that the sterilization conditions continue to be met. Temperatures should be recorded by independent measuring equipment.

16.27 Prepare a production load known to present the greatest challenge to the operating cycle and for which there is a PQ report. (This will normally be the reference load used in the yearly PRQ tests.)

16.28 Place the load in the chamber as described in the PQ report with temperature sensors in the following positions:

a. one (sensor A) in thermal contact with the sensor connected to the chamber temperature recorder;

b. one (sensor B) in thermal contact with the sensor connected to the chamber temperature indicator;

c. one in the item of the load which is the slowest to attain the sterilization temperature.

16.29 Where the chamber is pressurised during the cooling stage, connect a pressure recorder to measure the differential pressure across the air filter.

16.30 Ensure that the operating cycle corresponds with that used for the performance qualification test for the load. Start the cycle.

16.31 During the cooling stage, measure the differential pressure across the air filter.

16.32 The test should be considered satisfactory if the requirements listed in the PQ report are met.

Thermometric test for a full load

16.33 This test will have been carried out by the manufacturer as a type test. It need be repeated only if the sterilizer fails to meet the requirements of the thermometric test for performance qualification (see paragraph 16.22).

16.34 The test is adapted from the former BS3421 (now withdrawn). Temperatures should be recorded by independent measuring equipment as described in Chapter 6. For chambers with more than two shelves, two or more cycles may be required to measure the temperature at all the required points.

16.35 The test load should comprise the largest number of open-topped glass jars, nominally 12 cm high and 6 cm in diameter, which can be placed in the usable chamber space subject to the following conditions:

a. the shelves should be of the type provided for use with the sterilizer. The number of shelves should be the maximum that can be placed in the chamber such that the distances between the top of each layer of jars and the surface above (shelf or roof of chamber) is not less than 3 cm. For the purposes of this test, it is permissible to arrange the shelves on temporary supports;

b. on each shelf the number of jars should be the maximum that can be placed in rows parallel to and at right angles to the front of the chamber with at least 1 cm separating jars in adjacent rows.

16.36 Place 100 ml of a suitable heat-stable, non-volatile liquid in each of the four jars at the corners of each shelf and in the jar nearest to the centre of each shelf. The remaining jars should be empty. Suitable liquids for this purpose are silicone oils which remain liquid under the conditions of the test. Alternative liquids may be used providing they have a similar thermal behaviour.

16.37 Place temperature sensors in the following positions:

a. one (sensor A) in thermal contact with the sensor connected to the chamber temperature recorder;

b. one (sensor B) in thermal contact with the sensor connected to the chamber temperature indicator;

c. one in the centre of the liquid in each of the jars.

16.38 Select a sterilization temperature of 160°C. Adjust the timer to give a holding time of at least 2½ h (this is longer than the recommended minimum). Start the cycle.

16.39 At the end of the cycle, examine the recording of the chamber temperature measured by sensor A:

a. determine the mean temperature during the first 30 min of the holding time. If the temperature at any time before the start of the holding time is higher than this mean, the difference between the maximum temperature attained and this mean is the overheat;

b. determine the mean temperature during a 30-min period commencing 120 min after the start of the holding time. The difference between this mean and the mean determined for the start of the holding time is the temperature drift during a 2 h period.

16.40 The test should be considered satisfactory if the following requirements are met:

a. the requirements of the automatic control test (see paragraph 16.7) are met;

b. the temperature overheat does not exceed 2°C;

c. the holding time determined from the measured temperatures is not less than that specified in Table 8;

d. during the holding time:

   (i) the measured temperatures are within the appropriate sterilization temperature band specified in Table 8;

   (ii) the recorded chamber temperature is within 1°C of the temperature measured by sensor A;

   (iii) the indicated chamber temperature is within 1°C of the temperature measured by sensor B;

   (iv) the temperatures measured by each sensor in the load are within 5°C of the temperature measured by sensor A;

   (v) the temperature measured by sensor A does not drift by more than 2°C over a 2-h period;

   (vi) the temperature measured by sensor A does not fluctuate by more than 1°C;

e. the total cycle time is within the performance class stated by the manufacturer.

17.0 LTS disinfectors and LTSF sterilizers

Introduction

17.1 This chapter contains detailed procedures for tests specific to machines designed to process loads by exposure to low-temperature steam (LTS disinfectors) or low-temperature steam and formaldehyde (LTSF sterilizers). Schedules, prescribing which tests are to be carried out and when, are set out in Chapter 4 (for validation tests) and Chapter 5 (for periodic tests).

17.2 Machines are usually designed for both LTS and LTSF. These processes have similar characteristics and a machine incapable of meeting the LTS requirements will not normally meet the LTSF requirements. Note that some LTSF machines expose the load to a series of pulses of sterilant rather than a continuous holding time.

17.3 Attention is drawn to the safety information presented in Chapter 1 and the detailed safety precautions discussed in Part 4.

Chamber overheat cut-out test

17.4 This test is designed to show that the overheat cut-out mechanisms for the chamber and jacket will prevent the temperature of the chamber walls and free space from exceeding 80°C. Where two temperature control mechanisms are fitted (for the jacket and the chamber) the test should be done twice, with each mechanism inactivated alternately.

17.5 Temperatures should be recorded by independent measuring equipment as described in Chapter 6. If an LTSF sterilizer is being tested, the LTS cycle should be selected. If an LTS cycle is not available, the primary material for generating formaldehyde should be replaced with an inert substitute (see paragraph 1.29). The chamber should be empty except for the usual chamber furniture.

17.6 Place 12 temperature sensors in the following positions:

a. one in an active chamber discharge (see paragraph 6.26);

b. five on each of the two chamber side walls (one at the approximate centre and four adjacent to the corner positions of the usable chamber space);

c. one on the plane of the usable chamber space (not on the wall) at a point nearest to the steam inlet port.

17.7 Inactivate the chamber or jacket temperature control in accordance with the manufacturer's instructions.

17.8 Select and start the LTS operating cycle.

17.9 The test should be considered satisfactory if the following requirements are met:

a. the cut-out device operates and causes the heat source to be isolated from the machine and the operating cycle to advance to the drying stage;

b. none of the measured temperatures exceeds 80°C;

c. at the end of the cycle the door remains locked and a fault is indicated.

Chamber wall temperature test

17.10 This test is designed to show that the air removal stage will not start until the chamber walls are heated to within 2°C of the selected operating temperature. If an LTSF sterilizer is being tested, the LTS cycle should be selected. If an LTS cycle is not available, the primary material for generating formaldehyde should be replaced with an inert substitute (see paragraph 1.29).

17.11 Temperatures should be recorded by independent measuring equipment as described in Chapter 6. The chamber should be empty except for the usual chamber furniture.

17.12 Place 12 temperature sensors in the positions described for the chamber overheat cut-out test (see paragraph 17.6).

17.13 Select and start the LTS operating cycle.

17.14 The test should be considered satisfactory if the following requirements are met:

a. the air removal stage of the operating cycle does not start until the temperatures measured by the 10 sensors attached to the chamber side walls are within 2°C of the selected operating temperature;

b. after the first 5 min of the holding time all the temperatures measured in the chamber are within –0°C + 5°C of the temperature measured in the active chamber discharge.

Thermometric test for a small load

17.15 If an LTSF sterilizer is being tested, the LTS cycle should be selected. If an LTS cycle is not available, the primary material for generating formaldehyde should be replaced with an inert substitute (see paragraph 1.29).

17.16 Temperatures and pressures should be recorded by independent measuring equipment as described in Chapter 6.

17.17 Place a standard test pack (see paragraph 7.27) in the chamber with the bottom of the pack supported 100–200 mm above the centre of the chamber base.

17.18 Place three temperature sensors in the following positions:

a. one in an active chamber discharge (see paragraph 6.26);

b. one at the approximate centre of the test pack (the wire from the sensor should be carefully arranged to prevent steam tracking along it);

c. one placed 50 ± 5 mm above the approximate centre of the upper surface of the test pack.

17.19 Connect a pressure recorder (or test gauge) to the chamber.

17.20 Select the LTS cycle. Ensure that the process temperature is set to 73°C (corresponding to a sterilization temperature of 71°C). Start the cycle.

17.21 If a test gauge is being used, measure and note the chamber pressure at the approximate mid-point of the holding time.

17.22 The test should be considered satisfactory if the following requirements are met:

a. the requirements of the automatic control test (see paragraph 12.13) are met;

b. the holding time, determined from the measured temperatures, is not less than that specified in Table 8;

c. during the holding time:

  (i) the measured temperatures are within the temperature band specified in Table 8;

  (ii) the temperature measured above the test pack is within 4°C of the temperature measured in the active chamber discharge;

  (iii) the temperature measured in the centre of the test pack is within 2°C of the temperature measured in the active chamber discharge;

  (iv) the indicated and recorded chamber temperatures are within 1°C of the temperature measured in the active chamber discharge;

  (v) the indicated and recorded chamber pressures are within 0.05 bar of the measured pressure;

d. for sterilizers using vacuum as the sole method of drying:

  (i) the duration of the drying stage is not less than 3 min;

  (ii) the chamber pressure at the end of the stage does not exceed 50 mbar absolute;

e. at the end of the cycle the sheets are sensibly dry.

Thermometric test for a full load

17.23 This test applies to LTS disinfection cycles only. It is not required when the machine is to be used solely with an LTSF sterilization cycle.

17.24 The load is made up of a standard test pack (see paragraph 7.27) and additional folded sheets designed to represent the maximum mass of textiles which may be processed in the machine, and is used to demonstrate that, at the levels at which cycle variables are set, rapid and even penetration of steam into the centre of a load occurs and disinfecting conditions are achieved.

17.25 Temperatures and pressures should be recorded by independent measuring equipment as described in Chapter 6.

17.26 Place a standard test pack within the chamber in a position identified by the manufacturer as the most difficult to disinfect. This will normally be in the approximate centre of the chamber. Load the rest of the usable chamber space with stacks of sheets as described for porous load sterilizers (see paragraphs 13.17, 13.20).

17.27 Place three temperature sensors in the following positions:

a. one in an active chamber discharge (see paragraph 6.26);

b. one at the approximate centre of the test pack (the wire from the sensor should be carefully arranged to prevent steam tracking along it);

c. one below the approximate centre of the top sheet of the test pack.

17.28 Connect a pressure recorder (or test gauge) to the chamber.

17.29 Ensure that the LTS operating cycle is set to an operating temperature of 73°C. Start the cycle.

17.30 If a test gauge is being used, measure and note the chamber pressure at the approximate mid-point of the holding time.

17.31 The test should be considered satisfactory if the following requirements are met:

a. the requirements of the automatic control test (see paragraph 12.13) are met;

b. during the holding time:

   (i) the measured temperatures are within the temperature band specified in Table 8;

   (ii) the temperature measured in the centre of the test pack is within 2°C of the temperature measured in the active chamber discharge;

c. at the end of the test the sheets are sensibly dry;

d. the total cycle time is within the performance class stated by the manufacturer.

Environmental formaldehyde vapour test

17.32 This test is designed to determine the concentration of formaldehyde vapour discharged into the environment from the chamber and test load at the end of an LTSF cycle. A gas monitoring instrument is required as specified in paragraphs 6.54–56.

17.33 Line two modular cardboard instrument trays (or similar), approximately 600 mm × 300 mm × 50 mm, with a 12-mm thickness of high-density, open-cell polyurethane foam.

17.34 Place two stainless steel rods, each 400 ± 2 mm long by 10 ± 0.5 mm in diameter, in each tray and fit the lids. If the trays are smaller than specified above, the rods may be 250 mm long.

17.35 Place the trays side by side in the centre of the chamber.

17.36 Select the LTSF operating cycle. Ensure that the concentration of formaldehyde used for the test is that to be used for the microbiological test for basic performance. Start the cycle.

17.37 At the end of the cycle, measure the concentration of formaldehyde gas discharged from the chamber when the door starts to open. The sample should be taken 80–120 mm in front of the gap at a height of 1.4–1.6 m. Continue to sample the gas for the next 15 min.

17.38 Determine the average concentration of gas over the 15-min period.

17.39 The test should be considered satisfactory if the atmospheric concentration of formaldehyde gas over the 15-min period does not exceed the short-term exposure limit specified in Table 1.

Microbiological test for basic performance

17.40 Since the efficacy of LTSF sterilization cannot be assured by the measurement of cycle variables, the only definitive performance test currently available for LTSF sterilizers is microbiological. This test is designed to demonstrate the distribution and penetration of formaldehyde gas within the chamber. Chemical indicators are used to give an early indication of the efficacy of gas penetration but by themselves are not sufficient to validate the sterilization process. See Chapter 7 for advice on the use of biological and chemical indicators.

17.41 Place 27 inoculated carriers in the chamber arranged on fine thread to the pattern shown in Figure 16. (If the usable chamber space is less than 200 l fewer carriers may be used. The authorised person will advise on this.) Place a chemical indicator alongside each of the inoculated carriers.

17.42 Place an inoculated carrier and a chemical indicator in each of four Line-Pickerill helices (see paragraph 7.51). Double-wrap two of the helices in paper bags (that is, bag in bag) conforming to BS6257.

17.43 Place the wrapped helices in diametrically opposite corners of the sterilizer chamber; one in the upper rear of the usable chamber space, and the other in the lower front. Place one unwrapped helix in the front half of the usable chamber space and one in the rear half. All these positions are shown in Figure 16.

17.44 Ensure that the cycle variables are set to the values specified by the manufacturer. The concentration of formaldehyde is normally 15 g m^{-3} of chamber volume per pulse which can be achieved by the vaporisation of 40 ml of formalin per cubic metre of chamber volume. Start the operating cycle.

17.45 At the end of the cycle, remove the inoculated carriers and chemical indicators from the chamber and the helices. Check that the chemical indicators show a uniform colour change. If so, place each of the inoculated carriers in a bottle of recovery medium, and incubate them with controls as described in the general procedure for microbiological tests (see paragraphs 7.63–75).

17.46 If the chemical indicators do not show a uniform colour change, then the test should be abandoned.

17.47 The test should be considered satisfactory if the requirements given in paragraph 7.72 are met.

17.48 The test should be performed two more times to ensure that similar results are obtained.

17.49 The test should be reported in the format shown in Figure 17.

Microbiological test for performance qualification

17.50 This test is designed to follow a thermometric test for performance qualification. The loading condition and operating cycle should be identical. Chemical indicators are used to give an early indication of the efficacy of gas penetration but by themselves are not sufficient to validate the sterilization process. See Chapter 7 for advice on the use of biological and chemical indicators.

17.51 Put an inoculated carrier and a chemical indicator together in each of the six load items that carried temperature sensors in the thermometric test. Place the items in as nearly as possible in the same positions they occupied in the thermometric test. Put a biological indicator and a chemical indicator together in a Line-Pickerell helix (see paragraph 7.51) and place the helix in a position known to be the most difficult to sterilize (normally the coolest part of the chamber).

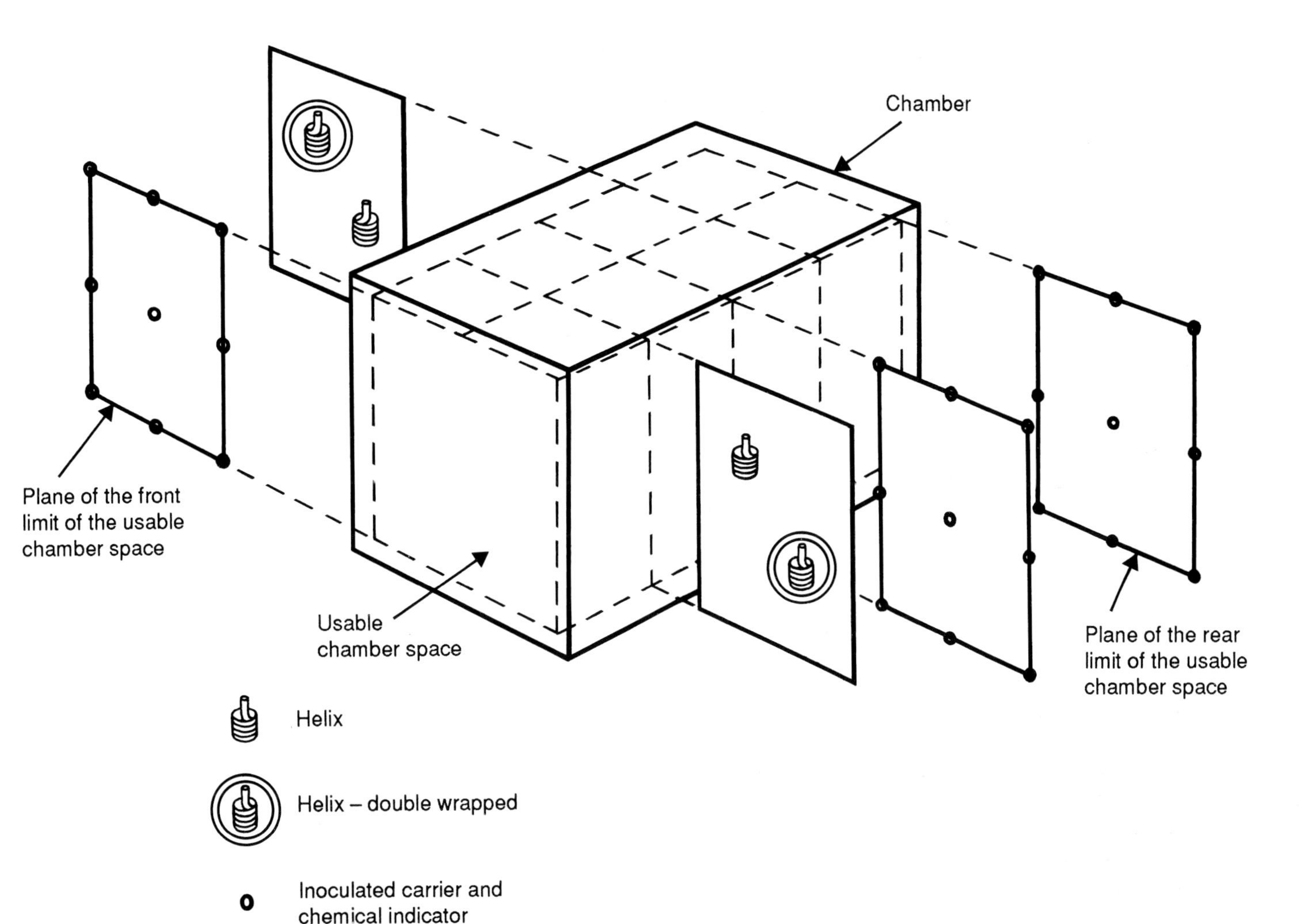

Figure 16 Layout of indicators for the microbiological test for basic performance (LTSF)

17.52 Select and start the operating cycle.

17.53 Ensure that a batch process record is made by the recording instrument fitted to the sterilizer.

17.54 At the approximate mid-point of the plateau period, note the elapsed time and indicated chamber temperature and pressure.

17.55 At the end of the cycle, remove the indicators from the load items and the helix. Check that the chemical indicators show a uniform colour change. If so, place each of the inoculated carriers in a bottle of recovery medium and incubate them with controls as described in the general procedure for microbiological tests (see paragraphs 7.63–75).

17.56 If the chemical indicators do not show a uniform colour change, then the test should be abandoned.

17.57 The test should be considered satisfactory if the following requirements are met:

a. during the whole of the cycle the values of the cycle variables as shown on the batch process record are within the permitted tolerances marked on the master process record established during the thermometric PQ test;

b. the requirements for microbiological tests set out in paragraph 7.72 are met.

LOW-TEMPERATURE STEAM AND FORMALDEHYDE STERILIZER
REPORT OF MICROBIOLOGICAL TEST FOR BASIC PERFORMANCE

Automatic controller settings for plateau period: Temperature ________ °C Time ________ min ________ s

Primary material for generating formaldehyde ____________ Batch no. ____________ Expiry date ____________

Mass of primary material used in the cycle: Setting ____________ gram Measured ____________ gram

CHEMICAL INDICATORS: Manufacturer ______________ Batch no.______________ Expiry date ______________

BIOLOGICAL INDICATORS: Manufacturer ______________ Organism ______________ Strain ______________

Manufacturer's declared number of recoverable spores on each indicator ____________

Batch no. ____________ Expiry date____________

LOCATIONS OF CHEMICAL AND BIOLOGICAL INDICATORS

Location	No	Chemical	Biological	No	Chemical	Biological	No	Chemical	Biological
Rear plane	1	PASS/FAIL	PASS/FAIL	2	PASS/FAIL	PASS/FAIL	3	PASS/FAIL	PASS/FAIL
	4	PASS/FAIL	PASS/FAIL	5	PASS/FAIL	PASS/FAIL	6	PASS/FAIL	PASS/FAIL
	7	PASS/FAIL	PASS/FAIL	8	PASS/FAIL	PASS/FAIL	9	PASS/FAIL	PASS/FAIL
Centre plane	10	PASS/FAIL	PASS/FAIL	11	PASS/FAIL	PASS/FAIL	12	PASS/FAIL	PASS/FAIL
	13	PASS/FAIL	PASS/FAIL	14	PASS/FAIL	PASS/FAIL	15	PASS/FAIL	PASS/FAIL
	16	PASS/FAIL	PASS/FAIL	17	PASS/FAIL	PASS/FAIL	18	PASS/FAIL	PASS/FAIL
Front plane	19	PASS/FAIL	PASS/FAIL	20	PASS/FAIL	PASS/FAIL	21	PASS/FAIL	PASS/FAIL
	22	PASS/FAIL	PASS/FAIL	23	PASS/FAIL	PASS/FAIL	24	PASS/FAIL	PASS/FAIL
	25	PASS/FAIL	PASS/FAIL	26	PASS/FAIL	PASS/FAIL	27	PASS/FAIL	PASS/FAIL
Line-Pickerell helices:			**Wrapped**	1	PASS/FAIL	PASS/FAIL	2	PASS/FAIL	PASS/FAIL
			Unwrapped	3	PASS/FAIL	PASS/FAIL	4	PASS/FAIL	PASS/FAIL

BIOLOGICAL CONTROLS

Unexposed BI	1	GROWTH/NO GROWTH	2	GROWTH/NO GROWTH	3	GROWTH/NO GROWTH
No BI	4	GROWTH/NO GROWTH	5	GROWTH/NO GROWTH	6	GROWTH/NO GROWTH

Test person: Name ______________________ **Signature** ______________________ **Date** ____________

Microbiologist: Name ______________________ **Signature** ______________________ **Date** ____________

Figure 17 Report of microbiological test for basic performance (LTSF)

Routine microbiological test

17.58 A routine microbiological test is required for every production load. Chemical indicators are used to give an early indication of the efficacy of gas penetration but by themselves are not sufficient to monitor the sterilization process. See Chapter 7 for advice on the use of biological and chemical indicators. Conditions under which the load may be released as sterile are discussed in Part 4.

17.59 Place an inoculated carrier and a chemical indicator in a Line-Pickerill helix (see paragraph 7.51). Double-wrap the helix in paper bags (that is, bag in bag) conforming to BS6257. Put it in the chamber with the normal production load.

17.60 Select and start the operating cycle.

17.61 At the end of the cycle, remove the inoculated carrier and chemical indicator from the helix. Check that the chemical indicator shows a uniform colour change. If so, place the inoculated carrier in a bottle of recovery medium and incubate it with controls as described in the general procedure for microbiological tests (see paragraphs 7.63–75).

17.62 If the chemical indicator does not show a uniform colour change, then the test should be abandoned.

17.63 The test should be considered satisfactory if the requirements for microbiological tests set out in paragraph 7.72 are met.

18.0 Ethylene oxide sterilizers

Introduction

18.1 This chapter contains detailed procedures for tests specific to sterilizers designed to process loads by exposure to ethylene oxide gas (EO). Schedules, prescribing which tests are to be carried out and when, are set out in Chapter 4 (for validation tests) and Chapter 5 (for periodic tests).

18.2 Attention is drawn to the safety information presented in Chapter 1 and the detailed safety precautions discussed in Part 4.

18.3 Humidity is the most critical cycle variable in EO sterilization but also the most difficult to measure and control. In several of these tests it is necessary to determine the humidity in the sterilizer chamber during the conditioning stage. The ideal method is to use humidity sensors calibrated for RH (see paragraphs 6.47–50), but if these are not available the RH should be calculated using the method given in Appendix 2. Because of the large errors in both methods, and the variation within the chamber, the new EN permits a relatively broad range of 40–85% RH and that is the value given here. Users should aim, however, to attain an ideal true value of 50–60% RH to ensure that no part of the chamber is allowed to reach the dangerous extremes of < 30% RH or > 95% RH.

Chamber overheat cut-out test

18.4 This test is designed to show that the overheat cut-out mechanisms for the chamber and jacket will prevent the temperature of the chamber free space from exceeding the gas exposure temperature by more than 6°C. Where cycles with different gas exposure temperatures are available, the test should be done for each cycle. Where two temperature control mechanisms are fitted (for the jacket and the chamber) the test should be done with each mechanism inactivated alternately.

18.5 The dimensions of the usable chamber space need to be known for this test. The space is assumed to be a rectangular box. If the usable chamber space is cylindrical, the planes referred to below are those of the smallest box that can contain it (see Figure 18).

18.6 Temperatures should be recorded by independent measuring equipment as described in Chapter 6. The chamber should be empty except for the usual chamber furniture. EO gas should be replaced with an inert substitute (see paragraph 1.29).

18.7 Place 12 temperature sensors in the following positions:

a. one in thermal contact with the sensor connected to the temperature recorder fitted to the sterilizer;

b. two on each of the planes of the usable chamber space, excluding doors (one at the approximate centre of the plane and one in a position known to be the hottest);

c. one on the plane of the usable chamber space at a point nearest to the steam inlet port.

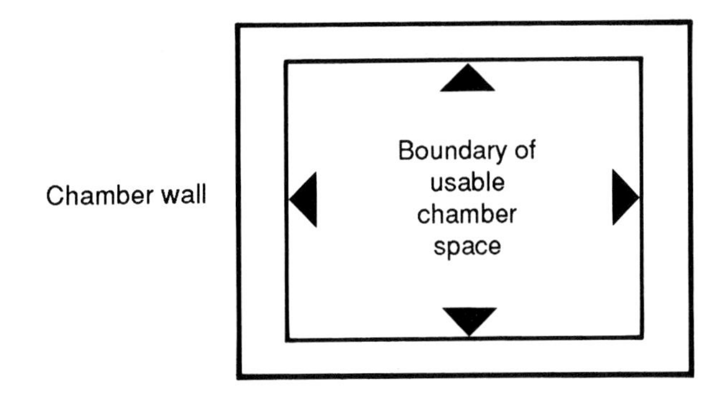

(a) Rectangular chamber

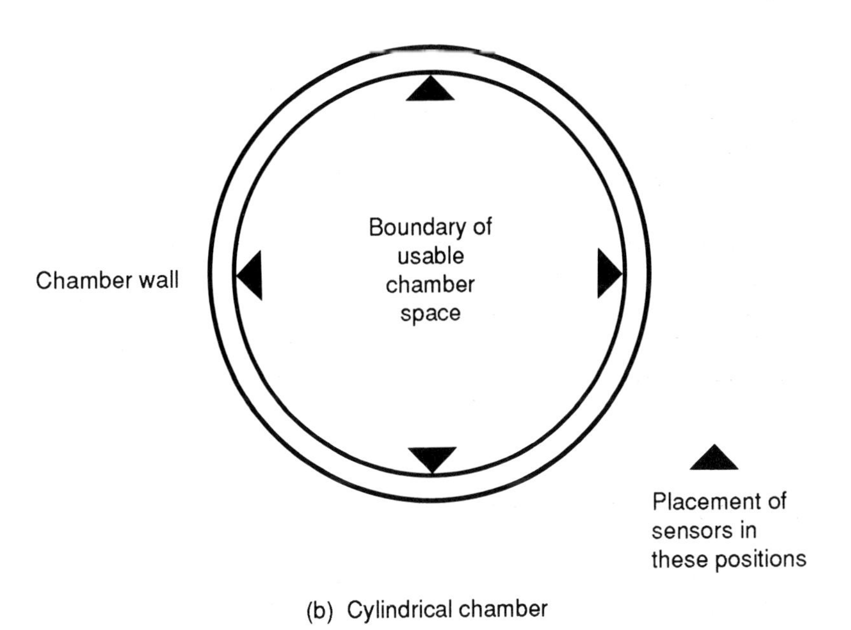

(b) Cylindrical chamber

Figure 18 Location of sensors for EO chamber overheat cut-out and chamber space temperature test

18.8 Inactivate the chamber or jacket temperature control in accordance with the manufacturer's instructions.

18.9 Select and start the operating cycle.

18.10 The test should be considered satisfactory if the following requirements are met:

a. the cut-out device operates and causes the heat source to be isolated from the machine and the operating cycle to advance to the gas removal stage;

b. none of the measured temperatures exceeds the preset gas exposure temperature by more than 6°C;

c. at the end of the cycle a fault is indicated.

Chamber space temperature test

18.11 This test is designed to show that the temperature of the chamber free space is within 2°C of the preset gas exposure temperature at the start of the gas exposure stage.

18.12 Temperatures should be recorded by independent measuring equipment as described in Chapter 6. The chamber should be empty except for the usual chamber furniture. EO gas should be replaced by an inert substitute (see paragraph 1.29).

18.13 Place 12 temperature sensors in the positions described for the chamber overheat cut-out test (see paragraph 18.7).

18.14 Select and start the operating cycle.

18.15 The test should be considered satisfactory if the following requirements are met:

a. at the start of the gas exposure stage the measured temperatures are within 2°C of the preset gas exposure temperature;

b. after the first 5 min of the gas exposure stage the temperatures measured in the chamber are within 2°C of the temperature measured by the sensor adjacent to the temperature recorder sensor.

Chamber wall temperature test

18.16 Temperatures should be recorded by independent measuring equipment as described in Chapter 6. The chamber should be empty except for the usual chamber furniture. EO gas should be replaced by an inert substitute (see paragraph 1.29).

18.17 Place 12 temperature sensors in the following positions:

a. one in thermal contact with the sensor connected to the temperature recorder fitted to the sterilizer;

b. two on each of the chamber surfaces, excluding doors (one at the centre of the surface and one in a position known to be the hottest);

c. one on the plane (not on the wall) of the usable chamber space at a point nearest to the steam inlet port.

18.18 Select and start the operating cycle.

18.19 The test should be considered satisfactory if, after the first 5 min of the gas exposure stage, the temperatures measured in the chamber are within 5°C of the temperature measured by the sensor adjacent to the temperature recorder sensor.

Microbiological test for gas exposure time

18.20 Since the efficacy of EO sterilization cannot be assured by the measurement of cycle variables, the only definitive performance test currently available for EO sterilizers is microbiological. This test is designed to demonstrate the penetration of EO gas within the chamber and to determine the duration of the gas exposure stage for routine production. Chemical indicators are used to give an early indication of the efficacy of gas penetration but by themselves are not sufficient to validate the sterilization process. See Chapter 7 for advice on the use of biological and chemical indicators.

18.21 During the conditioning stage it will be necessary to determine the relative humidity in the chamber. Humidity may be indicated or recorded by the instrument fitted to the sterilizer, calculated (Appendix 2) or referenced to a test in which an identical loading condition has been tested with an inert gas.

18.22 Place an inoculated carrier and a chemical indicator in each of four Line-Pickerill helices (see paragraph 7.51). Triple-wrap the helices in paper bags (that is, bag in bag in bag) conforming to BS6257. Seal the bags and allow them to equilibrate in an environment of 20 ± 5°C and 60 ± 20% RH for at least one hour.

18.23 Place two helices towards the front of the usable chamber space and two towards the rear, in positions known to be the slowest to attain the gas exposure temperature.

18.24 Select the operating cycle. The EO concentration in the chamber will normally be 250–1000 mg l^{-1}. The duration of the gas exposure stage should be considerably less than one-third of that anticipated for routine production, and insufficient to inactivate all the biological indicators. The authorised person will advise on what this period should be. Start the cycle.

18.25 At the end of the cycle remove the inoculated carriers and chemical indicators from the helices.

18.26 Repeat the cycle several times with fresh inoculated carriers and chemical indicators and the gas exposure time increased in each cycle. The gas exposure time for the final cycle should be sufficient to inactivate all the inoculated carriers. The behaviour of the chemical indicators may be used to estimate when this time is attained. The authorised person will advise on how many cycles are required and the time increment for each one.

18.27 Place each of the inoculated carriers in a bottle of recovery medium and incubate them with controls as described in the general procedure for microbiological tests (see paragraphs 7.63–7.75).

18.28 The test should be considered satisfactory if the following requirements are met;

a. at the end of the conditioning stage of each cycle the humidity in the chamber is in the range 40–85% RH (see paragraph 18.3);

b. at the end of the incubation period:

    (i) one or more of the bottles with inoculated carriers exposed to the EO process shows growth for the shortest gas exposure time, but none shows growth for the longest gas exposure time;

    (ii) control bottles with no inoculated carrier show no growth;

c. control bottles with unexposed inoculated carriers show growth within 24 h.

18.29 Note the shortest gas exposure time for which no growth is observed. Perform the test for a further two cycles at this exposure time. If all three cycles are satisfactory, the gas exposure time determined by this procedure (the critical gas exposure time) should be regarded as one-third of the minimum time required for production loads representing less of a challenge than the load used in this test.

Microbiological test for basic performance

18.30 This test is designed to demonstrate the penetration of EO gas within the chamber and confirm the duration of the gas exposure stage for routine production. Chemical indicators are used to give an early indication of the efficacy of gas penetration, but by themselves are not sufficient to validate the sterilization process. See Chapter 7 for advice on the use of biological and chemical indicators.

18.31 Prepare and position four Line-Pickerell helices as described in the microbiological test for gas exposure time (see paragraphs 18.22–18.23).

18.32 Select the operating cycle. Set the duration of the gas exposure stage to the critical gas exposure time determined during commissioning (see paragraph 18.29). Start the cycle.

18.33 At the end of the cycle remove the inoculated carriers and chemical indicators from the helices. Examine the chemical indicators and check whether they show a uniform colour change. If so, place each inoculated carrier in a bottle of recovery medium and incubate them with controls as described in the general procedure for microbiological tests (see paragraphs 7.63–7.75).

18.34 If the chemical indicators do not show a uniform colour change, then the test should be abandoned.

18.35 The test should be considered satisfactory if the following requirements are met:

a. at the end of the conditioning stage the humidity in the chamber is in the range 40–85% RH (see paragraph 18.3);

b. the requirements for microbiological tests set out in paragraph 7.72 are met.

Thermometric test for performance qualification

18.36 The load used for this test should be one of the production loads processed in the sterilizer. To serve as a reference load it should present to the process the greatest challenge on the basis of moisture absorbency, gas absorbency and the attainment of the gas exposure temperature throughout the load. If the load presents a greater challenge than the test load used in the microbiological test for basic performance, then that test will need to be repeated with the new load in order to confirm the gas exposure time.

18.37 Table 11 indicates the information that will need to be noted for the PQ report. See Chapter 8 for general information about PQ tests and reports.

18.38 Temperatures, pressures and humidities should be recorded by independent measuring equipment as described in Chapter 6. If humidity sensors are not available, humidity should be calculated as described in Appendix 2. EO gas should be replaced with an inert substitute (see paragraph 1.29).

18.39 Package each item of the load in accordance with the procedure to be used for routine production. Note the type of load and method of packaging.

18.40 Ensure that the preconditioning procedure is identical to that which will be used for production. This should normally be for at least 1 h in an environment having a temperature of 15–25°C and a humidity of 40–85% RH.

18.41 Place 12 temperature sensors in the following positions:

a. one in thermal contact with the sensor connected to the chamber temperature recorder fitted to the sterilizer (sensor A);

b. one in the gas entry port to the chamber;

The PQ report for EO sterilizers should include the values and permitted tolerances of the following variables:

1. *preconditioning (in separate area, if used):*
   a. time, temperature and humidity;
   b. minimum temperature of product permitted to enter preconditioning;
   c. maximum elapsed time between removal of the load from preconditioning and the start of the conditioning stage of the operating cycle;
2. *conditioning (in sterilizer chamber):*
   a. temperature and humidity in the chamber and within the load at the beginning and end of the conditioning stage;
   b. if a humidity indicator or recorder is not fitted to the sterilizer, the critical parameters necessary for the attainment of the specified humidity of the load – the parameters chosen will depend on the method used to humidify the load;
3. *sterilization:*
   a. chamber pressure;
   b. chamber temperature;
   c. gas exposure time;
   d. temperature of the load;
   e. EO concentration, estimated from pressure change (see Appendix 2) or (exceptionally) by direct analysis of chamber atmosphere;
4. *flushing (in sterilizer chamber):*
   a. time, temperature and pressure changes;
   b. rate of change of air or other gas;
   c. temperature of the load;
5. *degassing (in separate aeration cabinet and/or room):*
   a. Time, temperature and pressure changes;
   b. Rate of change of air or other gas;
   c. Temperature of the load.

Table 11 Performance qualification data for EO sterilizers

c. one in the primary heat source to the gas preheater (if fitted);

d. one in each of five load items known to be the slowest to attain the gas exposure temperature and placed in the coolest part of the chamber;

e. one in a load item in the hottest part of the chamber;

f. one in the coolest part of the chamber free space;

g. one on the hottest part of the chamber surface;

h. one on the coolest part of the chamber surface.

18.42 If available, place two humidity sensors in the following positions:

a. one alongside the temperature sensor in the load item in the hottest part of the chamber (see paragraph 18.41(e));

b. one alongside the temperature sensor in the coolest part of the chamber free space (see paragraph 18.41(f)).

18.43 Connect a pressure recorder (or test gauge) to the chamber.

18.44 Select the operating cycle that will be used for the production load. The cycle variables should be set as determined in the microbiological test for gas exposure time, although the duration of the flushing stage may need to be adjusted to satisfy the requirements of the environmental gas test (see paragraph 8.37) and the test for degassing time (see paragraph 8.46). Start the cycle.

18.45 Ensure that a batch process record is made by the recording instrument fitted to the sterilizer. This will serve as the basis for a master process record (see paragraph 8.58) for the loading condition under test.

18.46 At the end of the conditioning stage, note the readings from the humidity sensors, including the sterilizer humidity indicator (if fitted).

18.47 At the approximate mid-point of the gas exposure stage, note the elapsed time and the indicated chamber temperature and pressure.

18.48 The test should be considered satisfactory if the following requirements are met:

a. the requirements of the automatic control test (see paragraph 12.13) are met;

b. after the first 5 min of the gas exposure time the temperatures measured on the chamber walls are within 5°C of the temperature measured by sensor A;

c. after the first 5 min of the gas exposure time, and until its end, all the measured temperatures, except in the gas pre-heater and on the chamber walls, are within 2°C of the temperature measured by sensor A;

d. at the end of the conditioning stage:
   (i) the humidity is in the range 40–85% RH (see paragraph 18.3);
   (ii) the difference between the two RH measurements (if made) does not exceed 20% RH;
   (iii) the reading on the sterilizer humidity indicator (if fitted) is not less than 40% RH;

e. after the first 15 min of the gas exposure time, and until its end, the peak-to-peak variation in the measured chamber pressure does not exceed 20% for cylinder systems and 25% for cartridge systems;

f. for cylinder systems, throughout the cycle the temperature measured in the primary heat source to the gas pre-heaters does not exceed 70°C.

Microbiological test for performance qualification

18.49 This test is designed to follow a thermometric test for performance qualification. The loading condition, preconditioning process and operating cycle should be identical. Chemical indicators are used to give an early indication of the efficacy of gas penetration but by themselves are not sufficient to validate the sterilization process. See Chapter 7 for advice on the use of biological and chemical indicators.

18.50 Assemble 20 biological indicators and 20 chemical indicators to form 20 biological-chemical indicator pairs. Place them in the following positions:

a. one pair in each of the six load items which carried temperature sensors in the thermometric test (see paragraphs 19.41(d), (e));

b. 14 pairs distributed throughout the remaining load items.

18.51 Select the operating cycle used in the thermometric test. The concentration of EO used for the test should be the same as will be used for production cycles. This is normally 250–1000 mg l^{-1}. Start the cycle.

18.52 Ensure that a batch process record is made by the recording instrument fitted to the sterilizer.

18.53 At the end of the conditioning stage, note the indicated chamber temperature, pressure and humidity. Where a humidity instrument is not fitted, RH may be assumed to be the same as that determined during the thermometric test provided that all the cycle variables are identical within the permitted tolerances.

18.54 At the approximate mid-point of the gas exposure stage, note the elapsed time and the indicated chamber temperature, pressure and humidity.

18.55 At the end of the cycle, remove the indicators from the load items. Check whether the chemical indicators show a uniform colour change. If so, place each of the inoculated carriers in a bottle of recovery medium and incubate them with controls as described in the general procedure for microbiological tests (see paragraphs 7.63–7.75).

18.56 If the chemical indicators do not show a uniform colour change, then the test should be abandoned.

18.57 The test should be considered satisfactory if the following requirements are met;

a. the requirements of the automatic control test (see paragraph 12.13) are met;

b. the humidity values at the end of the conditioning stage, whether indicated, measured or calculated, are consistent with those obtained during the thermometric test;

c. the requirements for microbiological tests set out in paragraph 7.72 are met.

Routine microbiological test

18.58 A routine microbiological test is required for every production load. Chemical indicators are used to give an early indication of the efficacy of gas penetration but by themselves are not sufficient to monitor the sterilization process. See Chapter 7 for advice on the use of biological and chemical indicators. Conditions under which the load may be released as sterile are discussed in Part 4.

18.59 Assemble ten biological indicators and ten chemical indicators to form ten biological-chemical indicator pairs. Distribute the pairs evenly in the spaces between the load items.

18.60 Select and start the operating cycle.

18.61 At the end of the cycle, remove the indicators from the load. Check that the chemical indicators show a uniform colour change. If so, place each of the inoculated carriers in a bottle of recovery medium and incubate them with controls as described in the general procedure for microbiological tests given in Chapter 7.

18.62 If the chemical indicators do not show a uniform colour change, then the test should be abandoned.

18.63 The test should be considered satisfactory if the requirements for microbiological tests set out in paragraph 7.72 are met.

19.0 Laboratory sterilizers

Introduction

19.1 This chapter contains detailed procedures for tests specific to laboratory sterilizers. Schedules, prescribing which tests are to be carried out and when, are set out in Chapter 4 (for validation tests) and Chapter 5 (for periodic tests). The tests in this chapter apply to laboratory sterilizers equipped with one or more of the following operating cycles:

a. make-safe of small plastic discard;

b. make-safe of contained fluid discard;

c. sterilization of culture media (preset or variable cycle);

d. disinfection of fabrics (see paragraph 13.7 for the small-load test);

e. sterilization of glassware and equipment;

f. free steaming;

g. culture media preparator.

19.2 Attention is drawn to the safety information presented in Chapter 1 and the detailed safety precautions discussed in Part 4.

19.3 Unless specified otherwise, all the tests should be performed at each of the sterilization temperatures available on the sterilizer.

Make-safe of small plastic discard

19.4 These tests apply to laboratory sterilizers with an operating cycle designed to make-safe plastic discard material where no one item contains more than 50 ml of aqueous fluid.

19.5 If by agreement with the laboratory safety officer, the user authorises the use of the sterilizer with the thermal door-lock override selected, then these tests should be conducted both with and without the override selected.

Information about Hazard Groups may be found in the HSC document 'Categorisation of pathogens according to hazard and categories of containment' (second edition, 1990) compiled by the Advisory Committee on Dangerous Pathogens.

19.6 Containers should be held in the discard boxes recommended by the manufacturer. Discard boxes holding containers into which temperature sensors are to be inserted should not contain infected material. Material infected with Hazard Group 2 organisms may be used to make up other boxes in the test load. At no time should any material known to contain Hazard Group 3 or 4 organisms be used.

Thermometric test for a full load

19.7 Temperatures and pressures should be recorded by independent measuring equipment as described in Chapter 6.

19.8 Prepare sufficient Petri dishes to fill two discard boxes when the dishes are stacked vertically. Each dish should contain approximately 15 ml of agar gel.

19.9 Place one temperature sensor in the centre of each of six of the dishes. Put three of these test dishes in each box: one in the centre of the box, one

one-third from the bottom and one one-third from the top, supported by the remaining dishes. If only one box will fit in the chamber, put all six test dishes in the box, two at each position.

19.10 Put the two test boxes in opposite corners of the chamber. Load the remaining chamber space with boxes filled with discard material such that the spacing between boxes is in accordance with the minimum recommended by the manufacturer.

19.11 Place a further five temperature sensors in the following positions:

a. one in an active chamber discharge (see paragraph 6.26);

b. one in the chamber, alongside the sensing element of the load temperature probe, if it is fitted (the probe should be stowed on its bracket);

c. one in the centre of the free space between the bottom of each test box and its trivet (if fitted). (If the box does not have a trivet, the sensor should be placed in the free space between Petri dishes 15 mm above the centre of the bottom of the box);

d. one in the chamber free space.

19.12 Connect a pressure recorder (or test gauge) to the chamber.

19.13 Select and start the operating cycle.

19.14 If a test gauge is being used, measure the chamber pressure at the approximate mid-point of the holding time.

19.15 The test should be considered satisfactory if the requirements listed in Table 12 are met, and the drain is not blocked with agar.

Thermometric test for a small load

19.16 This test is not required if the sterilizer is designed to accommodate only one discard box. Temperatures and pressures should be recorded by independent measuring equipment as described in Chapter 6.

19.17 Load the chamber with a single discard box filled with Petri dishes as described in the full-load test, with three temperature sensors located in the following positions:

a. one in an active chamber discharge (see paragraph 6.26);

b. one in the centre of a dish located one-third from the bottom of the box;

c. one in the centre of a dish located in the approximate centre of the box.

19.18 Follow the procedure for the full-load test.

19.19 The test should be considered satisfactory if all but the cycle time condition of the requirements for the full-load test are met.

Cycles for fluid loads

19.20 These tests apply to laboratory sterilizers with cycles designed to process fluid discard in glass containers and large plastic containers (> 50 ml), culture media (preset or variable cycles) and for free steaming.

The test should be considered satisfactory if the following requirements are met:

a. the requirements of the automatic control test (paragraph 12.13) are met;

b. the holding time, as determined from the measured temperatures, is not less than that specified for the appropriate sterilization temperature band listed in Table 12;

c. during the holding time:

   (i) the measured temperatures are within the appropriate sterilization temperature band listed in Table 12;

   (ii) except for discard cycles, the measured temperatures are within 1°C of each other;

   (iii) the indicated and recorded chamber temperatures are within 1°C of the temperature measured in the active chamber discharge;

   (iv) the indicated and recorded chamber pressures are within 0.05 bar of the measured chamber pressure;

   (v) the measured chamber pressure is within 0.05 bar of saturated steam pressure or, if a partial pressure system is used, as specified by the manufacturer;

d. at the end of the cycle:

   (i) the temperature sensors have remained in position;

   (ii) items holding sensors remain intact;

   (iii) not more than one of the other items (or 1%, whichever is the greater) has burst or broken;

   (iv) the temperature measured in any fluid containers is not greater than 90°C (plastic) or 80°C (glass);

e. the total cycle time is within the performance class stated by the manufacturer.

Table 12 General requirements for the full-load test (laboratory sterilizers)

19.21 Bottles into which temperature sensors are inserted should contain a solution of 10–15 g of agar powder dissolved in 1000 ml of distilled water. Other bottles in the loads should be filled with water or water-based culture medium.

19.22 All bottles should be filled to 80% of their nominal capacity. The volumes of the fluid in each bottle should not vary from their mean by more than 5%. At the start of the cycle the temperature of the fluid in each bottle should be 20 ± 5°C and the media preparation in the liquid form.

19.23 The bottles may be either all sealed or all unsealed, according to the practice in the laboratory and the requirements of the schedules in Chapters 4 and 5. Sealed and unsealed bottles should not be mixed in the same load.

Thermometric test for a full load

19.24 Temperatures and pressures should be recorded by independent measuring equipment as described in Chapter 6.

19.25 Fill nine one-litre bottles with the test liquid as described in paragraph 19.21. Insert a temperature sensor into each one, ensuring that the tops are sealed or unsealed as required. Unsealed bottles should be capped loosely to prevent coolant water entering the bottle.

19.26 If unsealed bottles are used, weigh each of them and note their masses (M_1) to an accuracy of 1 g.

19.27 Place three of the bottles in positions known to be the slowest to attain the sterilization temperature, three in positions known to be the fastest to attain the sterilization temperature, and three in positions known to be the slowest to cool to 80°C.

19.28 Load the remaining chamber space with one-litre bottles, filled either with water or a water-based medium, at the minimum spacing recommended by the manufacturer.

19.29 Place a further temperature sensor in an active chamber discharge (see paragraph 6.26).

19.30 Connect a pressure recorder (or test gauge) to the chamber.

19.31 Select the operating cycle:

a. if a variable culture media cycle is being tested, set the sterilization temperature to 121°C with a minimum holding time of 15 min;

b. if a free steaming cycle is being tested, set the load temperature to 95–98°C for a minimum of 15 min.

19.32 Start the cycle.

19.33 If a test gauge is being used, measure the chamber pressure at the approximate mid-point of the holding time.

19.34 As soon as the cycle is complete, and before opening the door, observe and note the measured temperatures in the bottles.

19.35 Within 5 min of the end of the cycle, weigh any unsealed test bottles again and note their masses (M_2). For each bottle, calculate the percentage loss in mass from:

$$\text{Percentage loss in mass} = 100 \times \frac{(M_1 - M_2)}{M_1}$$

19.36 The test should be considered satisfactory if the requirements listed in Table 12 are met and the loss of fluid in any unsealed bottles does not exceed 2% by mass.

Thermometric test for a small load

19.37 Temperatures and pressures should be recorded by independent measuring equipment as described in Chapter 6.

19.38 Fill nine 5-ml bijou bottles with 4 ml of test liquid as described in paragraph 19.21. Insert a temperature sensor into each one, ensuring that the tops are sealed.

19.39 Distribute them among two wire baskets, one supported in the upper rear of the usable chamber space and the other in the lower front. Each should contain a total of 25 bijou bottles, so that three test bottles are in positions known to be the slowest to attain the sterilization temperature, three in positions known to be the fastest to attain the sterilization temperature, and three in positions known to be the slowest to cool to 80°C.

19.40 If the sterilizer is not designed to process bottles of this size, the smallest size and number of containers recommended by the sterilizer manufacturer should be used.

19.41 Where the sterilizer is to be used to process one size of container only, the test load may be a single container of this size, filled with the nominal volume of test liquid and supported in a position known to be the slowest to attain the sterilization temperature.

19.42 Place a further temperature sensor in an active chamber discharge (see paragraph 6.26).

19.43 Connect a pressure recorder (or test gauge) to the chamber.

19.44 Follow the procedure for the full-load test.

19.45 The test should be considered satisfactory if, except for the cycle time condition, the requirements listed in Table 12 are met.

Simplified thermometric test for performance requalification

19.46 This test is not a substitute for a full PRQ test, but is used quarterly to check that the sterilization conditions continue to be met. Temperatures and pressures should be recorded by independent measuring equipment as described in Chapter 6.

19.47 Prepare a production load known to present the greatest challenge to the operating cycle and for which there is a PQ report. (This will normally be the reference load used in the yearly PRQ tests.) Place temperature sensors in the following positions:

a. one in an active chamber discharge (see paragraph 6.26);

b. one in a container known to be the slowest to attain the sterilization temperature;

c. one in a container known to be slowest to cool to 80°C.

19.48 Place the load in the chamber as described in the PQ report.

19.49 Select the operating cycle as specified in the PQ report. Start the cycle.

19.50 The test should be considered satisfactory if the requirements listed in the PQ report are met.

Sterilization of glassware and equipment

19.51 These tests apply to laboratory sterilizers with a cycle designed to sterilize empty glassware without caps and other non-porous equipment. If caps are fitted, air will not be removed, and the glassware should be classed as disinfected but not sterilized.

Thermometric test for a full load

19.52 Temperatures and pressures should be recorded by independent measuring equipment as described in Chapter 6.

19.53 Fill four discard boxes with empty glass bijou bottles, without caps, arranged randomly. Place two temperature sensors in each box, one inserted into an inverted bottle in the centre of the box and one in an inverted bottle one-third from the bottom.

19.54 Where the full load is less than four boxes, the maximum load which the sterilizer is designed to process should be used. The eight temperature sensors should be distributed within the load.

19.55 Put these test boxes in the chamber and load the remaining chamber space with boxes of bijou bottles at the minimum spacing recommended by the manufacturer.

19.56 Place three further temperature sensors in the following positions:

a. one in an active chamber discharge (see paragraph 6.26);

b. one in the chamber located alongside the load temperature probe (if fitted);

c. one in the upper chamber free space.

19.57 Connect a test pressure recorder (or a test gauge) to the chamber.

19.58 Select and start the operating cycle.

19.59 If a test gauge is being used, measure the chamber pressure at the approximate mid-point of the holding time.

19.60 The test should be considered satisfactory if the requirements listed in Table 12 are met, and the load is visibly dry.

Thermometric test for a small load

19.61 Fill one discard box with bijou bottles with sensors placed as described for the full-load test and put it in the chamber. Place a further sensor in an active chamber discharge.

19.62 Follow the procedure for the full-load test.

19.63 The test should be considered satisfactory if, except for the cycle time condition, the requirements listed for the full-load test are met.

Thermal door-lock override test

19.64 A thermal door-lock is fitted to certain laboratory sterilizers to prevent the door from being opened until the temperature in the chamber and load falls below 80°C. The override is intended for use by trained persons who wish to gain access at temperatures above 80°C to loads which will not present an explosive hazard.

19.65 For this test the sterilizer chamber should be empty.

19.66 Select and start the operating cycle to be tested.

19.67 Attempt to select the thermal door-lock override during the heat-up, sterilization (holding time) and cooling stages.

19.68 The test should be considered satisfactory if the following requirements are met:

a. the override operates only during the cooling stage of the cycle and causes the cooling stage to terminate;

b. the override switch resets automatically when released;

c. the thermal door-lock override indicator is illuminated;

d. at the end of the cycle the door cannot be opened except by means of a key, code or tool which is unique to the sterilizer.

19.69 Where the sterilizer is intended to be used exclusively for make-safe of discard in small containers, compliance with (b) and (d) may be waived by agreement with the laboratory safety officer. In this case, the switch should reset automatically whenever a different operating cycle is selected or whenever the power supply is interrupted.

Culture media preparator

19.70 For these tests, the sterilizer vessel should be filled with the test liquid described in paragraph 19.21 to the nominal capacity specified by the manufacturer.

Thermometric test for a full load

19.71 Temperatures and pressures should be recorded by independent measuring equipment as described in Chapter 6.

19.72 Place two temperature sensors in the following positions:

a. one at the bottom of the chamber in the space occupied by the minimum production volume stated by the manufacturer;

b. one in the approximate centre of the chamber.

19.73 Connect a pressure recorder (or test gauge) to the chamber.

19.74 Select and start the operating cycle.

19.75 If a test gauge is being used, measure the chamber pressure at the beginning, middle and end of the holding time.

19.76 When the cycle is complete, wait for the temperature in the chamber to fall to 85°C. Attempt to open the door safety hood. If the hood does not open, wait for the temperature to fall below 80°C. Attempt to open the hood again.

19.77 The test should be considered satisfactory if the following requirements are met:

a. the requirements of the automatic control test (see paragraph 12.13) are met;

b. the holding time, as determined from the measured temperatures, is not less than that specified for the appropriate sterilization temperature band listed in Table 13;

c. during the holding time:

   (i) the temperatures measured in the medium are both within ± 2°C of the set temperature;

   (ii) the indicated and recorded chamber temperatures are within 1°C of the lower of the two temperatures measured in the medium;

   (iv) the indicated and recorded chamber pressures are within 0.05 bar of the measured chamber pressure;

d. the door safety hood cannot be opened until the higher of the two temperatures measured in the medium falls below 80°C.

Name of operating cycle	Sterilization temperature [°C]	Maximum temperature [°C]	Minimum holding time [min]
Make-safe of small plastic discard	134	138	3
	126	129	10
	121	124	15
Make-safe of contained fluid discard	134	138	3
	126	129	10
	121	124	15
Sterilization of culture media (pre-set cycle)	121	124	15
	115	118	30
Sterilization of culture media (variable cycle)	102–134		up to 60
	121[a]	124	15
Disinfection of fabrics	134	138	3
	126	129	10
	121	124	15
Sterilization of glassware and equipment	134	138	3
	126	129	10
	121	124	15
Free steaming (variable cycle)	102–104		up to 60
	95[a]	98	15
Culture media preparator	121	124	15
	115	118	30

a. Although the cycle is variable, this temperature band should be used for testing purposes.

Table 13 Sterilization conditions for laboratory sterilizers

Reheat and dispensing test

19.78 This test follows immediately after the full-load test, using the same load. Temperature and pressure sensors should be removed.

19.79 Set the sterilizer to reheat the batch to a nominal reheat temperature of 100°C.

19.80 Five minutes after the medium attains the reheat temperature, allow it to cool to a nominal dispensing temperature of 55°C.

19.81 When the indicated chamber temperature reaches 55°C wait 10 min and begin dispensing the medium.

19.82 Note the indicated chamber temperature and pressure at the beginning, middle and end of the dispensing period.

19.83 The test should be considered satisfactory if the following requirements are met:

a. during dispensing:
   - (i) the indicated chamber temperature is within ± 2°C of the set dispensing temperature;
   - (ii) the indicated chamber pressure is zero;
   - (iii) the medium does not solidify;
b. the person conducting the test does not observe any mechanical or other anomaly.

Glossary

The following list of definitions has been adopted in HTM 2010 and used in Part 3. Paragraph references indicate where further information may be found in Part 3. Cross-references to other terms are shown in bold type.

absolute pressure	Pressure measured from absolute vacuum.
active chamber discharge	The controlled flow of air, or of air and condensate, from the **chamber**, through either a drain or a vent, such that the temperature of the discharge is at the temperature of the chamber (see paragraph 6.26).
aeration	A part of the **sterilization process** during which **sterilant gas** and/or its reaction products desorb from the **load** until predetermined levels are reached. See **degassing** and **flushing**.
air detector	A device used to determine that sufficient air or other **non-condensable gases** have been removed from the **chamber** (see paragraph 11.37).
automatic controller	A device that, in response to predetermined **cycle variables**, operates the **sterilizer** sequentially through the required stages of the **operating cycle**.
automatic control test	A test designed to show that the **operating cycle** functions correctly as evidenced by the values of the **cycle variables indicated** and **recorded** by the instruments fitted to the **sterilizer** (Chapter 12).
A-weighted	Of sound level measurements, weighted to the frequency response of the human ear (see paragraph 10.2).
batch process record (BPR)	A permanent record of one or more **cycle variables recorded** during a complete **operating cycle** by instruments fitted permanently to the **sterilizer**.
biological indicator	A device, consisting of an **inoculated carrier** contained within a primary pack, designed to test the efficacy of an **operating cycle** (see paragraph 7.43).
cartridge	In **EO sterilizers**, a portable, single-use, simple vessel containing **sterilant** gas under pressure from which the gas is delivered by puncturing the cartridge.
chamber	The part of the **sterilizer** in which the **load** is placed.
chamber furniture	Shelves, pallets, loading trolleys and other fixed or movable parts that support the **load** within the **chamber**.
chamber temperature	The lowest temperature prevailing in the **chamber**.
chemical indicator	A device designed to show, usually by a change of colour, whether specified values of one or more **cycle variables** have been attained (see paragraph 7.36).
clinical sterilizer	A **sterilizer** designed to process **medical devices** to be used in the clinical care of patients.
commissioning	The process of obtaining and documenting evidence that equipment has been provided and installed in accordance with the equipment specifications and that it functions within predetermined limits when operated in accordance with the operational instructions (see paragraph 2.15).
conditioning	In **EO sterilizers**, the treatment of a **load** within the **operating cycle**, but prior to **sterilization**, to attain a predetermined temperature and humidity throughout the load.
cooling stage	The period of the **operating cycle**, after the **holding time** has been completed, during which the **load** remains in the **chamber** while the load cools to a safe temperature.

critical gas exposure time	For **EO sterilizers**, the shortest **gas exposure time**, determined during **commissioning**, for which all **biological indicators** are inactivated (see paragraph 18.20).
culture media preparator	A specialised **laboratory sterilizer** designed for the **sterilization** and dispensing of culture media.
cycle complete	Recognition by the **automatic controller** that the pre-set values for the **cycle variables**, necessary for a successful **operating cycle**, have been attained and that the sterilized **load** is ready for removal from the **chamber**.
cycle variables	The physical properties, for example time, temperature, pressure, humidity and gas concentration, that influence the efficacy of the **operating cycle** (see paragraph 7.3).
degassing	In **LTSF** and **EO sterilizers**, an **aeration** procedure in which **sterilant** gas and its reaction products are desorbed from the **load** by defined treatment outside the **sterilizer** after completion of the **operating cycle**.
disinfection	A process used to reduce the number of viable micro-organisms in a **load** but which may not necessarily inactivate some viruses and bacterial spores.
disinfector	An apparatus designed to achieve **disinfection**.
dry-heat sterilizer	A **clinical sterilizer** designed to sterilize **loads** by exposure to hot dry air at near atmospheric pressure.
dryness value	A dimensionless quantity, approximating to the dryness fraction, derived to determine whether steam is of the correct dryness for **sterilization** purposes. A dryness value of 1.0 represents **dry saturated steam** (see paragraph 9.30).
D-value	Decimal reduction value (for **biological indicators**). The time in minutes required to secure inactivation of 90% of the test organisms under stated exposure conditions.
EO sterilizer	A **clinical sterilizer** designed to sterilize **loads** by exposure to **EO** gas or EO gas mixtures.
equilibration time	The period which elapses between the attainment of the **sterilization temperature** in the **chamber** and the attainment of the sterilization temperature in all parts of the **load** (see paragraph 7.10).
ethylene oxide (EO)	**Sterilant** gas used to sterilize items that would be damaged by exposure to heat or moisture. Chemical formula CH_2CH_2O.
F_0	A quantity, measured in minutes, used to determine the efficacy of an **operating cycle** and equivalent to a continuous period at a temperature of 121°C (see paragraph 14.19).
fail-safe	An attribute of **sterilizer** design whereby failure of any component or its associated services does not create a safety hazard.
fault	The recognition by the **automatic controller** that the preset **cycle variables** for the **operating cycle** have not been attained, and that **sterilization** or **disinfection** has been jeopardised.
fluid sterilizer	A **clinical sterilizer** designed to sterilize fluids in sealed containers by exposure to **high-temperature steam** under pressure.
flushing	In **LTSF** and **EO sterilizers**, an **aeration** procedure by which remaining **sterilant** gas is removed from the **load** within the **chamber** by the passage of air or other inert gas.
formaldehyde	**Sterilant** gas used in combination with **low-temperature steam** to sterilize items that would be damaged by exposure to **high-temperature steam**. Chemical formula HCHO.
formalin	Formaldehyde solution BP. A 38% aqueous solution of **formaldehyde** stabilised with 10% w/v ethanol, commonly used as the primary material for generating formaldehyde gas.

free steaming	A process, used in **laboratory sterilizers**, in which the **load** is exposed to steam near atmospheric pressure.
full load	A specified **load**, used in thermometric tests, to represent the maximum size and mass of load which the **sterilizer** is designed to process (see paragraph 2.45).
gas exposure time	In **EO sterilizers**, the time for which the **chamber** is maintained at the specified temperature, gas concentration, pressure and humidity (see paragraph 18.20).
gauge pressure	Pressure measured from atmospheric pressure.
high-temperature steam	Steam at a temperature above the boiling point of water at local atmospheric pressure.
holding time	The period during which the temperature in all parts of the **chamber**, **load** and any coolant fluid is held within the **sterilization temperature band**. It follows immediately after the **equilibration time** (see paragraph 7.8).
hot-air sterilizer	See **dry-heat sterilizer**.
hot source	A temperature reference used to verify the calibration of a thermometric measurement system (see paragraph 6.33).
indicated	An indicated value is that shown by a dial or other visual display fitted permanently to the **sterilizer** (see **recorded** and **measured**) (see paragraph 7.3).
inoculated carrier	A component of a **biological indicator**, comprising a piece of supporting material on which a defined number of test organisms are deposited (see paragraph 7.44).
installation checks	A series of checks performed by the contractor to establish that the **sterilizer** has been provided and installed correctly, is safe to operate, does not interfere with nearby equipment and that all connected services are satisfactory and do not restrict the attainment of conditions for **sterilization** (see paragraph 2.17).
installation tests	A series of tests performed by the contractor after the **installation checks** to demonstrate that the **sterilizer** is working satisfactorily (see paragraph 2.20).
Köch steamer	A laboratory apparatus designed to expose a **load** to steam at near atmospheric pressure and commonly used for melting solidified agar.
laboratory sterilizer	A **sterilizer** designed to sterilize, disinfect or **make-safe** laboratory materials and equipment.
Line-Pickerell helix	A device containing an **inoculated carrier**, used in microbiological tests on **LTSF** and **EO sterilizers**, and designed to simulate the worst-case conditions for **sterilization** by gas (see paragraph 7.51).
load	Collectively, all the goods, equipment and materials that are put into a **sterilizer** or **disinfector** at any one time for the purpose of processing it by an **operating cycle**.
load item	One of several discrete containers, packs or other units that together constitute a **load**.
load temperature probe	A movable temperature sensor fitted within the **sterilizer chamber** and designed to record the temperature inside selected **load items**.
loading area	The room or area in front of the **sterilizer** in which the operator works and from which the sterilizer is loaded and unloaded. It is commonly separated by a fascia panel from the **plantroom**.
loading condition	A specified combination of the nature and number of **load items**, the items of **chamber furniture**, and their distribution within the **chamber** (see paragraph 8.7).
low-temperature steam (LTS)	Steam at a temperature below the boiling point of water at local atmospheric pressure.
LTS disinfector	A clinical **disinfector** designed to disinfect **loads** by exposure to **low-temperature steam** at sub-atmospheric pressure.

LTSF sterilizer	A **clinical sterilizer** designed to sterilize **loads** by exposure to **low-temperature steam** and **formaldehyde** gas at sub-atmospheric pressure.
make-safe	A process, used in **laboratory sterilizers**, to reduce the microbial content of contaminated material so that it can be handled and disposed of without causing an infection hazard or environmental contamination.
master process record (MPR)	A **batch process record** obtained from a thermometric **commissioning** or **performance qualification** test and annotated to show the **permitted tolerances** for **cycle variables** during subsequent testing and routine production (see paragraph 8.58).
measured	A measured value is that shown on a test instrument, such as a thermometric recorder or a test pressure gauge, attached to the **sterilizer** for test purposes (see **indicated** and **recorded**) (see paragraph 7.6).
medical device	Any instrument, apparatus, appliance, material or other article, whether used alone or in combination, including the software necessary for its proper application intended by the manufacturer, to be used for human beings for the purpose of: diagnosis, prevention, monitoring, treatment or alleviation of disease; diagnosis, monitoring, treatment, alleviation of or compensation for an injury or handicap; investigation, replacement or modification of the anatomy or of a physiological process; and control of conception: and which does not achieve its principal intended action in or on the human body by pharmacological, immunological or metabolic means, but which may be assisted in its function by such means. (Source: EU Council Directive 93/42/EEC)
medicinal product	Any substance or combination of substances presented for treating or preventing disease in human beings or animals. Any substance or combination of substances which may be administered to human beings or animals with a view to making a medical diagnosis or to restoring, correcting or modifying physiological functions in human beings or in animals is likewise considered a medicinal product. (Source: EU Council Directive 65/65/EEC)
non-condensable gases	Gases which cannot be liquefied by compression under the range of conditions of temperature and pressure used during the **operating cycle** (see paragraph 9.4).
noted	A noted value is that written down by the operator, usually as the result of observing an **indicated**, **recorded** or **measured** value (see paragraph 7.7).
operating cycle	The set of stages of the **sterilization** or **disinfection** process carried out in sequence and regulated by the **automatic controller**. It is synonymous with the terms "sterilization cycle" for **sterilizers** and "disinfection cycle" for **disinfectors**.
override	A system by which the progress of the **operating cycle** can be interrupted or modified as necessary.
performance class	An integer, from 1 to 12, related to the total cycle time for a **sterilizer** with a **full load**.
performance qualification (PQ)	The process of obtaining and documenting evidence that the equipment, as commissioned, will produce an acceptable product when operated in accordance with the process specification (see paragraph 2.25).
performance requalification (PRQ)	The process of confirming that the evidence obtained during **performance qualification** remains valid (see paragraph 8.64).
periodic tests	A series of tests carried out at daily, weekly, quarterly and yearly intervals (see paragraph 2.36).
permitted tolerance	A limit, determined during **performance qualification**, on how much a **cycle variable** is permitted to vary from a nominal value (see paragraph 8.47).
plant history file	A file containing **validation**, maintenance and other engineering records for each **sterilizer**.

plantroom	The room or area to the rear of the **sterilizer** in which services are connected and which provides access for maintenance. It is commonly separated by a fascia panel from the **loading area**.
plateau period	The **equilibration time** plus the **holding time** (see paragraph 7.11).
porous load sterilizer	A **clinical sterilizer** designed to process, by exposure to **high-temperature steam** under pressure, porous items such as towels, gowns and dressings, and also **medical devices** that are wrapped in porous materials such as paper or fabrics.
PQ report	A report containing the data and results obtained from a **performance qualification** test (see paragraph 8.54).
preconditioning	Treatment of a **load** to attain predetermined conditions, such as temperature and humidity, before the start of an **operating cycle**.
pressure vessel	A collective term describing the sterilizer **chamber**, jacket (if fitted), door(s) and components that are in permanent open connection with the chamber.
recommissioning	A procedure to confirm that operational data established during **commissioning** remain valid (see paragraph 2.39).
recorded	A recorded value is that shown on the output of a recording instrument fitted permanently to the **sterilizer** (see **indicated** and **measured**) (see paragraph 7.5).
reference load	A specified **load** made up to represent the most difficult combination of items to be sterilized (see paragraph 8.7).
repeat validation	A procedure to obtain a new set of **commissioning** and **performance qualification** data to replace the set originally obtained during **validation** (see paragraph 2.41).
revalidation	A procedure to confirm an established **validation**, consisting of **recommissioning** followed by **performance requalification** (see paragraph 2.39).
safety hazard	A potentially detrimental effect on persons or the surroundings arising directly from either the **sterilizer** or its **load**.
saturated steam	Steam whose temperature, at any given pressure, corresponds to that of the vaporisation curve of water.
small load	A specified **load**, used in thermometric tests, to represent the minimum size and mass of load which the **sterilizer** is designed to process (see paragraph 2.45(a)).
standard test pack	A pack representing the maximum density of porous material which a **porous load sterilizer** conforming to European Standards should be able to process (see paragraph 7.27).
sterilant	An agent used to effect **sterilization**, such as steam, hot air or a sterilizing gas.
sterile	Condition of a **load item** that is free from viable micro-organisms. See EN 556 for the requirements for a **medical device** to be labelled "sterile".
sterilization	A process undertaken to render a **load sterile**.
sterilization conditions	The ranges of the **cycle variables** which may prevail throughout the **chamber** and **load** during the **holding time** (see paragraph 7.8).
sterilization pressure band	The range of pressures which may prevail in the **chamber** during the **holding time**. For a steam **sterilizer**, the sterilization pressure band is directly related to the **sterilization temperature band**.
sterilization process	The complete set of procedures required for **sterilization** of a **load**, including the **operating cycle** and any treatment of the load before or after the operating cycle.
sterilization temperature	Minimum acceptable temperature of the **sterilization temperature band** (see paragraph 7.14).
sterilization temperature band	The range of temperatures which may prevail throughout the **load** during the **holding time**. These temperatures are expressed as a minimum acceptable (the

	sterilization temperature) and a maximum allowable, and are stated to the nearest degree Celsius (see paragraph 7.14).
sterilizer	An apparatus designed to achieve **sterilization**.
sterilizer process log	A log, kept by the user, which contains records of each production cycle.
superheated steam	Steam whose temperature, at any given pressure, is higher than that indicated by the vaporisation curve of water.
thermal door-lock	An interlock fitted to certain **sterilizers** to prevent the door from being opened until the temperature in the **chamber** and **load** falls below a preset value (see paragraph 19.64).
transportable	Requiring no permanent connections or installation and capable of being moved manually without mechanical assistance. Synonymous with "bench-top".
type tests	A series of tests conducted by the manufacturer to establish the working data for a **sterilizer** type (see paragraph 2.11).
usable chamber space	The space inside the **chamber** which is not restricted by **chamber furniture** and which is consequently available to accept the **load**.
validation	A documented procedure for obtaining, recording and interpreting data required to show that a **sterilization process** will consistently comply with predetermined specifications (see paragraph 2.14).
working pressure	The pressure in the **chamber** during the **plateau period** of an **operating cycle**.
works tests	A series of tests to establish the efficacy of each **sterilizer** at the manufacturer's works (see paragraph 2.11).

Abbreviations

ATCC	American Type Culture Collection
BPR	batch process record
BS	British Standard
CEN	European Committee for Standardisation (Comité Européen de Normalisation)
CIP	Collection Institut Pasteur (France)
COSHH	Control of Substances Hazardous to Health (Regulations)
dBA	decibel, A-weighted
EMF	electromotive force
EN	European Standard (Europäische Norm)
EO	ethylene oxide
EU	European Union (formerly European Community)
h	hour(s)
HSC	Health and Safety Commission
HSE	Health and Safety Executive
HTM	Health Technical Memorandum
l or *l*	litre(s)
LTEL	long-term exposure limit
LTS	low-temperature steam
LTSF	low-temperature steam and formaldehyde
m	minute(s)
MPR	master process record
NCIMB	National Collections of Industrial and Marine Bacteria (UK)
NCTC	National Collection of Type Cultures (US)
ppm	parts per million
PQ	performance qualification
PRQ	performance requalification
RH	relative humidity
s	second(s)
SSD	sterile services department
STEL	short-term exposure limit
UK	United Kingdom

Bibliography

Unless stated otherwise, all the publications listed below are available from HMSO Books, 59 Nine Elms Lane, London SW8 5DR; tel 071 873 0011 (general enquiries), 071 873 0022 (order enquiries), (0800) 282827 (free information line); fax 071 873 8463.

Legislation

The Active Implantable Medical Devices Regulations 1992 (SI 1992/3146), ISBN 0 11 025389 2.

The Control of Substances Hazardous to Health Regulations 1988 (SI 1988/1657), ISBN 0 11 0867657 1.

The Pressure Systems and Transportable Gas Containers Regulations 1989 (SI 1989/2169), ISBN 0 11 098169 3.

European Union Directives

('*OJEC*' = *Official Journal of the European Communities*)

65/65/EEC – Council Directive of 26 January 1965 on the approximation of provisions laid down by law, regulation or administrative action relating to proprietary medicinal products, *OJEC*, No 22, p 369 (9 Feb 1965).

90/385/EEC – Council Directive of 20 June 1990 on the approximation of the laws of the Member States relating to active implantable medical devices, *OJEC*, No L189, p 17 (20 Jul 1990).

93/42/EEC – Council Directive of 14 June 1993 concerning medical devices, *OJEC*, No L169, p 1 (12 Jul 1993).

Health and safety publications

Health and Safety Commission (HSC) and Health and Safety Executive (HSE) publications are available from HSE Books, PO Box 1999, Sudbury, Suffolk CO10 6FS. General enquiries and requests for free leaflets should be addressed to the HSE Information Centre, Broad Lane, Sheffield S3 7HQ; tel (0742) 892345 (general enquiries), (0742) 892346 (free leaflets); fax (0742) 892333.

Advisory Committee on Dangerous Pathogens, **Categorisation of pathogens according to hazard and categories of containment** (second edition) (HSE, 1990), ISBN 0 11 885564 6.

Health Services Advisory Committee, **Safe working and the prevention of infection in clinical laboratories** (HSC, 1991), ISBN 0 11 885446 1.

Health Services Advisory Committee, **Safe working and the prevention of infection in clinical laboratories: model rules for staff and visitors** (HSC, 1991), ISBN 0 11 885442 9.

Occupational Exposure Limits (EH40), HSE (published annually).

British Standards

British Standards are available from the Sales Department, British Standards Institution, Linford Wood, Milton Keynes MK14 6LE; tel (0908) 226888 (enquiries), (0908) 221166 (orders); fax (0908) 322484.

BS593: 1989 Specification for laboratory thermometers

BS1780: 1985 (1992) Specification for bourdon tube pressure and vacuum gauges (AMD 6124, Jul. 1989)

BS1781: 1981 (1989), Specification for linen and linen union textiles

BS1904: 1984, Specification for industrial platinum resistance thermometer sensors (AMD 5671, Sep 1987; AMD 7049, Jun 1992)

BS2646: Autoclaves for sterilization in laboratories:

- **Part 1: 1993, Specification for design, construction, safety and performance**
- **Part 2: 1990, Guide to planning and installation**
- **Part 3: 1993, Guide to safe use and operation**
- **Part 4: 1991, Guide to maintenance**
- **Part 5: 1993, Methods of test for function and performance**

BS2775: 1987 (1992), Specification for rubber stoppers and tubing for general laboratory use

BS3693: 1992, Recommendations for design of scales and indexes on analogue indicating instruments (AMD 7448, Feb 1993)

BS3970: Sterilizing and disinfecting equipment for medical products:

- **Part 1: 1990, Specification for general requirements**
- **Part 2: 1991, Specification for steam sterilizers for aqueous fluids in sealed rigid containers**

Part 3: 1990, Specification for steam sterilizers for wrapped goods and porous loads

Part 4: 1990, Specification for transportable steam sterilizers for unwrapped instruments and utensils

Part 5: 1990, Specification for low-temperature steam disinfectors

Part 6: 1993, Specification for sterilizers using low-temperature steam with formaldehyde

BS4196: Sound power levels of noise sources:

Part 6: 1981 (1986), Survey method for determination of sound power levels of noise sources

BS4937: International thermocouple reference tables:

Part 4: 1973 (1981), Nickel-chromium/nickel-aluminium thermocouples, Type K (AMD 3986, Jun 1982)

Part 5: 1974 (1981), Copper/copper-nickel thermocouples, Type T (AMD 3987, Jun 1982)

BS5164: 1975 (1993), Specification for indirect acting electrical indicating and recording instruments and their accessories

BS5295: Environmental cleanliness in enclosed spaces:

Part 1: 1989, Specification for clean rooms and clean air devices (AMD 6602, Dec 1990)

BS5750: Quality systems (several parts)

BS5815: Sheets, sheeting, pillowslips, towels, napkins, counterpanes and continental quilt secondary covers for use in the public sector:

Part 1: 1989, Specification for sheeting, sheets and pillowslips (AMD 6806, Dec 1991)

BS6257: 1989, Specification for paper bags for steam sterilization for medical use

BS6447: 1984, (1992) Specification for absolute and gauge pressure transmitters with electrical outputs (AMD 5223, Sep 1986)

BS6698: 1986, Specification for integrating-averaging sound level meters (AMD 6323, Jun 1991)

BS7720: 1994, Specification for non-biological sterilization indicator systems equivalent to the Bowie and Dick test

European Standards

European Standards (issued in the UK with the prefix BS EN) are available from the British Standards Institution (address above). The titles of draft standards* may change before publication.

EN 285:* Sterilization – steam sterilizers – large sterilizers

EN 290:* Steam sterilizers – large sterilizers – terminology

EN ???:* Sterilizers for medical purposes – ethylene oxide sterilizers – specification

EN ???:* Small steam sterilizers

EN 550:* Sterilization of medical devices: validation and routine control of sterilization by ethylene oxide

EN 554:* Sterilization of medical devices: validation and routine control of sterilization by moist heat

EN 556:* Sterilization of medical devices: requirements for medical devices to be labelled "STERILE"

EN 837: Pressure gauges:

Part 1:* Bourdon tube pressure gauges – Dimensions, metrology, requirements and testing

EN 866: Biological systems for testing sterilizers:

Part 1:* General requirements

Part 2:* Systems for use in ethylene oxide sterilizers

Part 3:* Systems for use in steam sterilizers

Part 5:* Systems for use in low-temperature steam and formaldehyde sterilizers

Part 6:* Systems for use in dry-heat sterilizers

EN 867: Non-biological systems for use in sterilizers:

Part 1:* General requirements

Part 2:* Process indicators (Class A)

Part 3:* Specification for Class B indicators for use in the Bowie and Dick test

EN 30993: Biological evaluation of medical devices:

Part 7:* Ethylene oxide sterilization residuals

EN 60584: Thermocouples:

Part 2: 1993, Tolerances

EN 61010: Safety requirements for electrical equipment for measurement, control and laboratory use:

Part 1: 1993, General requirements

Part 2–041:* Particular requirements for autoclaves and sterilizers using steam for the treatment of medical materials and for laboratory processes

Part 2–042:* Particular requirements for autoclaves and sterilizers using toxic gas for the treatment of medical materials and for laboratory processes

??? – number not yet assigned

Department of Health publications

Department of Health publications are available from HMSO (address above).

Bacteriological tests for graded milk (Memo 139/ Foods) (Ministry of Health, January 1937)

Health Building Notes

Sterile services department (HBN 13) (NHS Estates, 1992), ISBN 0 11 321412 X

Accommodation for pathology services (HBN 15) (NHS Estates, 1991), ISBN 0 11 321401 4

Health Technical Memoranda

Sterilizers (HTM 10) (DHSS, 1980) (out of print)

Other references

JH Bowie, JC Kelsey and GR Thomson, **The Bowie and Dick autoclave tape test**, *Lancet*, **16**, 586–587 (1963)

SJ Line and JK Pickerell, **Testing a steam-formaldehyde sterilizer for gas penetration efficiency**, *Journal of Clinical Pathology*, **26**, 716–720 (1973)

JM Parry, PCB Turnbull and JR Gibson, **A colour atlas of bacillus species**, (Wolfe Medical Publications, 1983), ISBN 0 7234 0777 0 (hbk), 0 7234 1557 9 (pbk)

Appendix 1

Useful addresses

UK health agencies

NHS Estates, 1 Trevelyan Square, Boar Lane, Leeds LS1 6AE; tel (0532) 547000

Medicines Control Agency, Market Towers, 1 Nine Elms Lane, London SW8 5NQ; tel 071 273 3000

Medical Devices Agency, 14 Russell Square, London WC1B 5EP; tel 071 972 2000

NHS in Scotland Management Executive, St Andrew's House, Edinburgh EH1 3DG; tel 031 556 8400

Welsh Office, Cathays Park, Cardiff CF1 3NQ; tel (0222) 825111

Estate and Property Division, Estate Services Directorate, HPSS Management Executive, Stoney Road, Dundonald, Belfast BT16 0US; tel (0232) 520025

Public Health Laboratory Service, Central Public Health Laboratory, 61 Colindale Avenue, London NW9 5HT; tel 081 200 4400

Health and safety

Health and Safety Executive, Broad Lane, Sheffield S3 7HQ; tel (0742) 892345; fax (0742) 892333 (addresses of area HSE offices may be found in the local telephone directory)

Standards organisations

British Standards Institution

Head office: 2 Park Street, London W1A 2BS
Publications: Linford Wood, Milton Keynes MK14 6LE; tel (0908) 221166

European Committee for Standardisation, rue de Stassart 36, B–1050 Brussels

Bacterial culture collections

American Type Culture Collection (ATCC), 12301 Park Lawn Drive, Rockville, Maryland 20852–1776, USA; tel +1 301 881 2600

Collection Institut Pasteur (CIP), Institut Pasteur, 25 rue du Roux, F–75724 Paris Cédex 15, France

National Collection of Type Cultures (NCTC), Central Public Health Laboratory, 61 Colindale Avenue, London NW9 5HT

National Collections of Industrial and Marine Bacteria Ltd (NCIMB), 23 St Machar Drive, Aberdeen AB2 1RY

Other organisations

Clinical Pathology Accreditation (UK) Ltd, Pathology Block, The Children's Hospital, Western Bank, Sheffield S10 2TH; tel (0742) 797472

Institution of Hospital Engineering, 2 Abingdon House, Cumberland Business Centre, Northumberland Road, Portsmouth PO5 1DS; tel (0705) 823186

Appendix 2 Calculations

Derivation of the steam dryness value equation

A2.1 The equation given in Chapter 9 for the steam dryness value can be derived as follows.

A2.2 Steam supplied from the main will contain dry steam with a small amount of moisture carried as droplets in suspension at the same temperature. The dryness fraction, D, is defined as:

$$D = \frac{M_{dry}}{M_{steam}} = \frac{M_{dry}}{M_{dry} = M_{wet}} \qquad \text{(A2–1)}$$

where a given mass M_{steam} of steam contains a mass M_{dry} of pure dry steam and M_{wet} of moisture. Dry saturated steam has a dryness fraction of 1.0.

A2.3 If dry saturated steam is allowed to condense in cold water, then the temperature rise of the water is related to the amount of latent heat given up by the condensing steam. If the steam contains moisture, then the latent heat (and the temperature rise) will be less than for the same mass of pure dry saturated steam. The dryness fraction may then be estimated (the estimate being known as the dryness value) by equating the heat gained by the water to the heat lost by the steam.

A2.4 At the start of the test the flask contains a mass M_w of water at a temperature of T_0. At the end of the test the temperature has risen to T_1.

$$\text{Heat gained by water} = (T_1 - T_0)cM_w \qquad \text{(A2–2)}$$

where c is the specific heat capacity of water at a representative temperature between T_0 and T_1.

A2.5 The heat lost by the steam is equal to the latent heat of condensation plus the heat lost from the condensate and moisture as they cool from T_s to T_1.

$$\text{Heat lost by steam} = LM_{dry} + (T_s - T_1)cM_c = DLM_c + (T_s - T_1)cM_c \qquad \text{(A2–3)}$$

where L is the specific latent heat of condensation of steam at temperature T_s and $M_c = M_{steam}$ is the mass of condensate and moisture. Equating (A2–2) and (A2–3) and solving for D gives:

$$D = \frac{(T_1 - T_0)(cM_w + A)}{LM_c} - \frac{(T_s - T_1)c}{L} \qquad \text{(A2–4)}$$

where the term A represents the effective heat capacity of the flask and other apparatus. For the apparatus specified in Chapter 9, A can be taken as 0.24 kJ K^{-1} (see Table A1). If the apparatus being used differs significantly from Table A1 then the effective heat capacity should be recalculated.

A2.6 *Example*: In a dryness value test the temperature of the water in the flask rises from T_1 = 19°C to T_2 = 81°C. The average steam temperature during this time is T_s = 144°C. The initial mass of water in the flask is M_w = 632 g, and the mass of condensate is M_c = 77 g. From tables $c \approx 4.18$ kJ kg^{-1} K^{-1}, and $L \approx$ 2130 kJ kg^{-1}. Then:

$$D = \frac{(81 - 19)(4.18 \times 0.632 + 0.24)}{2130 \times 0.077} - \frac{(144 - 81)4.18}{2130} = 1.089 - 0.124 \approx \mathbf{0.96}.$$

Component[a]	Mass [g]	Heating factor[b]	Effective heat capacity [kJ K^{-1}]
One-litre glass vacuum flask	355	0.5	0.119
Rubber bung	91	0.8	0.116
90-mm glass pipe	2.4	1.0	0.002
290-mm glass pipe	7.8	1.0	0.005
TOTAL			0.242

a. The rubber pipe is not included as it is assumed to be at steam temperature at the start of the test.

b. The heating factor is an estimate of the factor by which the component is heated from T_1 to T_2 during the test.

Table A1 Effective heat capacity for steam dryness apparatus

A2.7 It can be seen that the term for the heat capacity of the apparatus (0.24) contributes approximately 10% to the total dryness value.

Relative humidity in EO sterilizers

A2.8 Due to the difficulty in measuring relative humidity in the chamber of an EO sterilizer, it is usually better to calculate the RH from the measured or recorded rise in pressure as humidifying steam is introduced.

A2.9 At the start of the conditioning stage the chamber contains a small amount of air at pressure P_0 and temperature T. During the conditioning stage steam is introduced into the chamber and the pressure rises to P_1 while the temperature remains at T. From the law of partial pressures we can identify the pressure change, $\Delta P = P_1 - P_0$, with the partial pressure of the water vapour, P_w.

A2.10 Relative humidity is defined as P_w/P_s where P_s is the saturated vapour pressure of water at temperature T, which can be obtained from steam tables. Hence,

$$\text{relative humidity, RH} = \Delta P/P_s \qquad \text{(A2–5)}$$

A2.11 *Example:* During a conditioning stage at a temperature of 55°C, the chamber pressure rises from P_0 = 80 mbar to P_1 = 168 mbar, a rise of ΔP = 88 mbar (8.8 kPa). From the steam tables we find that at 55°C, P_s = 157 mbar. The relative humidity is then 88/157 ≈ 0.56 = **56%**.

Concentration of ethylene oxide

A2.12 The concentration of ethylene oxide (EO) in a sterilizer chamber may be calculated as follows.

A2.13 An ideal gas obeys the equation of state:

$$Pv = \frac{Pm}{\rho} = RT \qquad \text{(A2–6)}$$

where:

P = absolute pressure (Pa);
v = molar volume (m^3 mol^{-1});
m = molecular weight (kg mol^{-1});
ρ = density (kg m^{-3});
R = gas constant (8.314 J K^{-1} mol^{-1});
T = absolute temperature (K).

A2.14 At the end of the conditioning stage, the chamber contains a mixture of air and water vapour at a pressure P_1 and temperature T. During the sterilant gas injection stage the pressure rises to P_2 while the temperature remains at T. From the law of partial pressures the pressure change, $\Delta P = P_2 - P_1$ can be identified with the partial pressure of the EO mixture:

$$\Delta P = P_{EO} + P_{DG} = RT \left(\frac{\rho_{EO}}{m_{EO}} + \frac{\rho_{DG}}{m_{DG}} \right) \quad \text{(A2–7)}$$

where the subscript EO refers to ethylene oxide and DG to the diluent gas. Rearranging for the EO density:

$$\rho_{EO} = m_{EO} \left(\frac{\Delta P}{RT} - \frac{\rho_{DG}}{m_{DG}} \right). \quad \text{(A2–8)}$$

A2.15 But from equation (A2.6):

$$\rho_{DG} = w_{DG}\rho = w_{DG} \frac{\Delta P \overline{m}}{RT} \quad \text{(A2–9)}$$

where $\overline{m}$ is the mean molecular weight of the EO mixture and w_{DG} is the proportion by mass of diluent gas such that $w_{EO} + w_{DG} = 1$.

A2.16 Inserting equation (A2–9) in equation (A2–8) gives the EO concentration:

$$\rho_{EO} = \frac{\Delta P}{RT} m_{EO} \left(1 - w_{DG} \frac{\overline{m}}{m_{DG}} \right). \quad \text{(A2–10)}$$

A2.17 The mean molecular weight of a mixture of two gases, 1 and 2, is defined as:

$$\overline{m} = \frac{n_1 m_1 + n_2 m_2}{n_1 + n_2} = \frac{\rho_1 + \rho_2}{\rho_1/m_1 + \rho_2/m_2} = \frac{(\rho_1 + \rho_2) m_1 m_2}{\rho_1 m_2 + \rho_2 m_1} = \frac{m_1 m_2}{w_1 m_2 + w_2 m_1} \quad \text{(A2–11)}$$

where n_1 and n_2 are the number of molecules of each gas. Hence, for an EO mixture the mean molecular weight is given by:

$$\overline{m} = \frac{m_{EO} m_{DG}}{w_{EO} m_{DG} + w_{DG} m_{EO}}. \quad \text{(A2–12)}$$

A2.18 Inserting equation (A2–12) in equation (A2–10) and rearranging, the concentration of EO in the chamber is:

$$\rho_{EO} = \frac{\Delta P}{RT} w_{EO} \overline{m}. \quad \text{(A2–13)}$$

A2.19 *Example:* A sterilizer uses a mixture of 12% EO (molecular weight: 44 g mol^{-1}) and 88% dichlorodifluoromethane (molecular weight: 121 g mol^{-1}). From equation (A2–12), the mean molecular weight of the mixture is then:

$$\overline{m} = \frac{44 \times 121}{0.12 \times 121 + 0.88 \times 44} = 100.0 \text{ g mol}^{-1}.$$

A2.20 During the gas injection stage the pressure is observed to rise by 1.48 bar (1.48×10^5 Pa) while the temperature remains at 55°C (328 K). From equation (A2–13) the concentration of EO in the chamber, in SI units, is then:

$$\rho_{EO} = \frac{1.48 \times 10^5 \times 0.12 \times 0.100}{8.31 \times 328} = 0.652 \text{ kg m}^{-3} \approx \mathbf{0.65\ g\ l^{-1}}.$$

A2.21 *Example:* A sterilizer uses a mixture of 10% EO and 90% carbon dioxide (molecular weight: 44 g mol^{-1}), giving an effective molecular weight of 44 (since both gases have the same molecular weight). During the gas injection stage the pressure rises by 5.16 bar (5.16×10^5 Pa) while the temperature remains at 37°C (310 K). From equation (A2–13) the concentration of EO in the chamber is then 0.881 kg m^{-3}, or **0.88 g l^{-1}**.

Appendix 3

Summary sheets

A3.1 The following summary sheets for commissioning, performance qualification and yearly or revalidation tests should be completed by the test person and given to the user as described in paragraph 2.30.

A3.2 They cover porous load sterilizers, fluid sterilizers, sterilizers for unwrapped instruments and utensils, dry-heat sterilizers, LTS disinfectors and LTSF sterilizers, EO sterilizers and laboratory sterilizers.

A3.3 The lists of tests are to be regarded as a record of which tests have been done, not a prescription for which tests ought to be done. Detailed schedules are given in Chapters 4 and 5. Tests which do not apply to the sterilizer under test should be marked "N/A".

A3.4 Where fluid or dry-heat sterilizers are to be used for the sterilization of medicinal products the sheets should be signed by the quality controller as shown.

A3.5 Common sheets are used for LTS and LTSF machines since most of the tests are identical. The signature of the microbiologist is required only for LTSF sterilizers.

A3.6 The sheets for laboratory sterilizers are designed to be used with any of the following operating cycles: make-safe of small plastic discard, make-safe of contained fluid discard, sterilization of culture media (preset or variable cycle), disinfection of fabrics, sterilization of glassware and equipment, free steaming. They may also be used for a culture media preparator. For commissioning and performance qualification, a separate sheet should be completed for each operating cycle available on the machine, and the name of the cycle written clearly in the space provided.

Reference ..../SC Page 1 of 2

POROUS LOAD STERILIZER - SUMMARY OF COMMISSIONING TESTS

Hospital .... Department .... Date(s) of tests ....

STERILIZER: Manufacturer .... Model .... Usable chamber space .... litres

Serial number .... Plant reference number ....

RESULT OF COMMISSIONING TESTS Data file reference ....

Test (as specified in HTM 2010 * = optional)	Pass or fail	Cycle number	Start time h min s	Results
Steam non-condensable gas	....			Concentration of NCG .... %
Steam superheat	....	....		Superheat ..... °C
Steam dryness	....	....		Dryness value ....
Automatic control	....	....	....	Sterilization temp (ST) selected ..... °C
Instrument calibration	....	....	....	See below
Chamber wall temperature	....	....	....	Max temp attained ..... °C
Air detector small load	....	....	....	Leak rate .... mbar/min
Air detector full load	....	....	....	Leak rate .... mbar/min
Thermometric full load	....	....	....	ST selected ..... °C Max temp ..... °C
Load dryness*	....	....	....	Average gain in mass ..... %
Thermometric small load	....	....		ST selected ..... °C Max temp ..... °C
Load dryness*	....	....	....	Average gain in mass ..... %
Vacuum leak (final)	....	....		Leak rate .... mbar/min
Hospital load dryness	....	....		
Air detector function	....	....		Air detector setting .... mbar or °C
Bowie-Dick	....	....		Type of test pack ....
Sound pressure*	....	....		Loading area: mean ..... dBA, peak ..... dBA
				Plant room: mean ..... dBA, peak ..... dBA

Test equipment file references ....

STERILIZER INSTRUMENT CALIBRATION

Errors for instruments fitted to sterilizer as measured by test instruments during the holding time.

Sensor is *measured reading - recorded/indicated error.*

	Measured	Recorder error	Indicator error
Chamber temperature	.... °C	.... °C	.... °C
Chamber pressure	.... bar	.... bar	.... bar

POROUS LOAD STERILIZER - SUMMARY OF COMMISSIONING TESTS

SUMMARY OF THERMOMETRIC TESTS

Sterilization temperature (ST) selected .... °C
Automatic controller settings for plateau period: Temperature .... °C Time .... min .... s

Event	Elapsed time		Chamber pressure	Temperature sensors		
	min	s	bar	Drain/ vent °C	Test pack °C	Free space °C
SMALL LOAD TEST				No	No	No .....
Start of plateau period	....	....	....	....	....	....
Start of holding time	....	....	....	....	....	....
End of holding time	....	....	....	....	....	....
Maximum values attained			....	....	....	....
Equilibration time	....	....				
Holding time	....	....				
Total cycle time	....	....				
FULL LOAD TEST				No	No	No .....
Start of plateau period	....	....	....	....	....	....
Start of holding time	....	....	....	....	....	....
End of holding time	....	....	....	....	....	....
Maximum values attained			....	....	....	....
Equilibration time	....	....				
Holding time	....	....				
Total cycle time	....	....				

DECLARATION OF TEST PERSON (STERILIZERS)

1. The installation checks and tests have been completed and show that the sterilizer has been provided and installed in accordance with its specifications.
2. All test instruments have current calibration certificates.
3. Calibration of the temperature test instruments has been checked before and after the thermometric tests.
4. The commissioning tests have been completed and show that the sterilizer functions correctly when operated in accordance with operational instructions.

Test Person: Name .... Signature .... Date ....

DECLARATION OF USER
The sterilizer is fit for use. The first yearly tests are due no later than :

User: Name .... Signature .... Date ....

Reference ..../SPQ Page 1 of 2

POROUS LOAD STERILIZER - SUMMARY OF PERFORMANCE QUALIFICATION TESTS

Hospital .... Department .... Date(s) of tests ....

STERILIZER: Manufacturer .... Model .... Usable chamber space ....litres

Serial number .... Plant reference number...

Chamber shape .... Width .... mm Height ....mm Depth ....m

OPERATING CYCLE REFERENCE .... Sterilization temperature ....°C

LOADING CONDITION REFERENCE .... Batch reference ....

Nature of load ....

LOCATION OF SENSORS FOR THERMOMETRIC PQ TEST

Enter positions of temperature sensors within the chamber related to the bottom left-hand corner of a rectangular box viewed from the loading end.

Sensor number	Sensor Type	Width (X) mm	Height (Y) mm	Depth (Z) mm	Location of sensor
1	T				Active chamber drain/vent
2	T				
3	T				
4	T				
5	T				
6	T				
7	T				
8	T				
9	T				
10	T				
11	T				
12	T				
13	P				Chamber pressure test port

(T = Temperature P = Pressure)

Test equipment file references ....

POROUS LOAD STERILIZER - SUMMARY OF PERFORMANCE QUALIFICATION TESTS

SUMMARY OF THERMOMETRIC PQ TEST

Sterilization temperature (ST) selected .... °C

Automatic controller setting for plateau period: Temperature .... °C Time .... min .... s

Identify sensors in the load which are the fastest and the slowest to attain the ST. Enter elapsed times and measured chamber pressures and temperatures.

Sensor number	Description	Sensor first attains ST		Sensor falls below ST		Time above ST	Max temp
		Time min s	Press bar	Time min s	Press bar	min s	°C
....	Drain/vent	....	....	....	....	....	....
....	Fastest	....	....	....	....	....	....
....	Slowest	....	....	....	....	....	....

Equilibration time ..... min ..... s Holding time ..... min ..... s Total cycle time ..... min ..... s

Cycle number .... Master Process Record reference ....

Is a microbiological PQ test required for this loading condition? ....

Result of microbiological test PASS/FAIL PQ report reference ....

DECLARATION OF TEST PERSON (STERILZERS)

1. This test has been preceded by a satisfactory sequence of commissioning/yearly tests. Reference ....
2. All test instruments have current calibration certificates.
3. Calibration of the thermometric test instruments has been verified before and after the thermometric tests.
4. The performance qualification tests show that the sterilizer produces acceptable product with the loading condition identified above.

Test Person: Name .... Signature .... Date ....

DECLARATION OF USER

The sterilizer is fit for use with the loading condition identified above. The first performance requalification test, due ....

User: Name .... Signature .... Date ....

Reference ..../SY Page 1 of 1

POROUS LOAD STERILIZER - SUMMARY OF YEARLY/REVALIDATION TESTS

Hospital .... Department .... Date (s) of tests ....

STERILIZER: Manufacturer .... Model .... Usable chamber space .... litres

Serial number .... Plant reference number ....

RESULTS OF YEARLY/REVALIDATION TESTS

Data file reference ....

Test (as specified in HTM 2010)	Pass or fail	Cycle number	Start time h min s	Results
Yearly safety checks	....			
Automatic control	....	....	....	Sterilization temp (ST) selected ..... °C
Instrument calibration	....	....	....	See below
Air detector small load	....	....	....	Leak rate .... mbar/min
Air detector full load	....	....	....	Leak rate .... mbar/min
Thermometric small load	....	....	....	ST selected ..... °C Max temp ..... °C
Vacuum leak (final)	....	....		Leak rate .... mbar/min
Air detector function	....	....		Air detector setting .... mbar or °C
Bowie-Dick	....	....		Type of test pack ....

PERFORMANCE REQUALIFICATION (if required)

PQ report reference	Loading condition ref	Operating cycle ref	ST °C	Thermometric: Pass or fail	Thermometric: Cycle number	Thermometric: Start time h min s	Microbio. (optional): Pass or fail	
....	....	....	....	....	....	....	....	
....	....	....	....	....	....	....	....	
....	....	....	....	....	....	....	....	

Test equipment file references ....

DECLARATION OF TEST PERSON (STERILIZERS)

1. All test instruments have current calibration certificates.
2. Calibration of the temperature test instruments has been checked before and after the thermometric tests.
3. The yearly/revalidation checks and tests have been completed and confirm that the sterilizer is safe to use and that commissioning and performance qualification data collected during validation remain valid.

Test Person: Name .... Signature .... Date ....

DECLARATION OF USER

The sterilizer is fit for use. The first yearly tests are due no later than :

User: Name .... Signature .... Date ....

Reference ..../SC

FLUID STERILIZER - SUMMARY OF COMMISSIONING TESTS

Hospital .... Department .... Dates(s) of tests ....

Sterilizer: Manufacturer .... Model .... Usable chamber space .... litres

Serial number .... Plant reference number ....

RESULTS OF COMMISSIONING TESTS

Data file reference ....

Test (as specified in HMT 2010 * = optional)		Pass or fail	Cycle number	Start time h min s	Results
Heat exchanger integrity					Test pressure .... bar
Automatic control					Sterilization temp (ST) selected .... °C
Instrument calibration					See below
Chamber temp profile					Max temperature attained .... °C
Thermometric small load					ST selected .... °C Max temp .... °C
					Decontamination time ..... min ..... s
Thermometric full load					ST selected ..... °C Max temp ..... s
					Decontamination time ..... min ..... s
Coolant quality					Concentration of residue .... mg/litre
Sound pressure*					Loading area:mean ... dBA, peak ... dBA
					Plant room: mean ... dBA, peak ... dBA

Test equipment file references ....

STERILIZER INSTRUMENT CALIBRATION

Errors for instruments fitted to sterilizer as measured by test instruments during the holding time.
Sense is measured reading = recorded/indicated error

	Measured	Recorder error	Indicator error
Chamber temperature	.... °C	..........°C	.... °C
Load temperature (1)	.... °C	..........°C	
Load temperature (2)	.... °C	..........°C	
Chamber pressure	.... bar	.... bar	.... bar

Reference ..../SC Page 2 of 2

FLUID STERILIZER - SUMMARY OF COMMISSIONING TESTS

SUMMARY OF THERMOMETRIC TESTS

Sterilization temperature (ST) selected .... °C
Automatic controller settings for plateau period: Temperature .... °C Time .... min .... s
Door release temperature setting .... °C Fo setting .... min

Event	Elapsed time		Chamber pressure	Spray pressure	Temperature sensors		
					Drain/	Fast	Slow
	min	s	bar	bar	vent °C	°C	°C
SMALL LOAD TEST					No	No	No .....
Start of plateau period	....	....	....	....	....	....	....
Start of holding time	....	....	....	....	....	....	....
End of holding time	....	....	....	....	....	....	....
Maximum values attained			....	....	....	....	....
Fo value at end					..... min	..... min	..... min
Equilibration time	....	....					
Holding time	....	....					
Total cycle time	....	....					

Temperature of hottest container when cycle complete .... °C (sensor no. .....)

Event	min	s	bar	bar	Drain/ vent °C	Fast °C	Slow °C
FULL LOAD TEST					No	No	No .....
Start of plateau period	....	....	....	....	....	....	....
Start of holding time	....	....	....	....	....	....	....
End of holding time	....	....	....	....	....	....	....
Maximum values attained			....	....	....	....	....
Fo value at end					..... min	..... min	..... min
Equilibration time	....	....					
Holding time	....	....					
Total cycle time	....	....					

Temperature of hottest container when cycle complete .... °C (sensor no. .....)

DECLARATION OF TEST PERSON (STERILIZERS)

1. The installation checks and tests have been completed and show that the sterilizer has been provided and installed in accordance with its specifications.
2. All test instruments have current calibration certificates.
3. Calibration of the temperature test instruments has been checked before and after the thermometric tests.
4. The commissioning tests have been completed and show that the sterilizer functions correctly when operated in accordance with operational instructions.

Test Person: Name .... Signature .... Date ....

DECLARATION OF USER AND FOR MEDICINAL PRODUCTS QUALIFIED PERSON

The sterilizer is fit for use. The first yearly tests are due no later than :

User: Name .... Signature .... Date ....

Qualified Person: Name .... Signature .... Date ....

Reference ..../SPQ Page 1 of 2

FLUID STERILIZER - SUMMARY OF PERFORMANCE QUALIFICATION TESTS

Hospital .... Department .... Date(s) of tests ....

STERILIZER: Manufacturer .... Model .... Usable chamber space ....litres

Serial number .... Plant reference number...

Chamber shape .... Width .... mm Height ....mm Depth ....m

OPERATING CYCLE REFERENCE .... Sterilization temperature ....°C

LOADING CONDITION REFERENCE .... Batch reference ....

Nature of load ....

LOCATION OF SENSORS FOR THERMOMETRIC PQ TEST

Enter positions of temperature sensors within the chamber related to the bottom left-hand corner of a rectangular box viewed from the loading end.

Sensor number	Sensor type	Width (X) mm	Height (Y) mm	Depth (Z) mm	Location of sensor
1	T				Active chamber drain/vent
2	T				
3	T				
4	T				
5	T				
6	T				
7	T				
8	T				
9	T				
10	T				
11	T				
12	T				
13	P				Chamber pressure test port
14	P				Spray pressure test port

(T = Temperature P = Pressure)

Test equipment file references ....

Reference ..../SPQ Page 2 of 2

FLUID STERILIZER - SUMMARY OF PERFORMANCE QUALIFICATION TESTS

SUMMARY OF THERMOMETRIC PQ TEST

Sterilization temperature (ST) selected .... °C

Automatic controller setting for plateau period: Temperature .... °C Time .... min .... s

Door release temperature setting .... °C F. setting .... min

Identify sensors in the load which are the fastest and the slowest to attain the ST. Enter elapsed times and measured chamber pressures and temperatures.

Sensor number	Description	Sensor first attains ST		Sensor falls below ST		Time above ST	Max temp	Fo
		Time min s	Press bar	Time min s	Press bar	min s	°C	min
....	Drain/vent	....	....	....	....	....	....	....
....	Fastest	....	....	....	....	....	....	....
....	Slowest	....	....	....	....	....	....	....

Equilibration time ..... min ..... s Holding time ..... min ..... s Total cycle time ..... min ..... s

Temp of hottest bottle at end .... °C (sensor .....) Coolant decontamination time ..... min ..... s

Cycle number .... Master Process Record reference ....

Is a microbiological PQ test required for this loading condition? ....

Result of microbiological test PASS/FAIL PQ report reference ....

DECLARATION OF TEST PERSON (STERILZERS)

1. This test has been preceded by a satisfactory sequence of commissioning/yearly tests.
   Reference ....
2. All test instruments have current calibration certificates.
3. Calibration of the thermometric test instruments has been verified before and after the thermometric tests.
4. The performance qualification tests show that the sterilizer produces acceptable product with the loading condition identified above.

Test Person: Name .... Signature .... Date ....

DECLARATION OF USER AND FOR MEDICINAL PRODUCTS QUALIFIED PERSON

The sterilizer is fit for use with the loading condition identified above. The first performance requalification test, due ....

User: Name .... Signature .... Date ....

Qualified Person: Name .... Signature .... Date ....

Reference ..../SY

FLUID STERILIZER - SUMMARY OF YEARLY/REVALIDATION TESTS

Hospital .... Department .... Date (s) of tests ....

STERILIZER: Manufacturer .... Model .... Usable chamber space .... litres

Serial number .... Plant reference number ....

RESULTS OF YEARLY/REVALIDATION TESTS

Data file reference ....

Test (as specified in HTM 2010)	Pass or fail	Cycle number	Start time h min s	Results
Yearly safety checks				
Heat exchanger integrity	....	....		Test pressure .... bar
Automatic control	....	....	....	Sterilization temp (ST) selected .... °C
Instrument calibration	....	....	....	See below
Coolant quality	....	....		Concentration of residue .... mg/litre

PERFORMANCE REQUALIFICATION

PQ report reference	Loading condition ref	Operating cycle ref	ST °C	Thermometric			Microbio. (optional)	
				Pass or fail	Cycle number	Start time h min s	Pass or fail	
....	....	....	....	....	....	....	....	
....	....	....	....	....	....	....	....	
....	....	....	....	....	....	....	....	
....	....	....	....	....	....	....	....	
....	....	....	....	....	....	....	....	

Test equipment file references ....

DECLARATION OF TEST PERSON (STERILIZERS) AND USER

1. All test instruments have current calibration certificates.
2. Calibration of the temperature test instruments has been checked before and after the thermometric tests.
3. The yearly/revalidation checks and tests have been completed and confirm that the sterilizer is safe to use and that commissioning and performance qualification data collected during validation remain valid.

Test Person: Name .... Signature .... Date ....

DECLARATION OF USER AND FOR MEDICINAL PRODUCTS QUALIFIED PERSON

The sterilizer is fit for use. The first yearly tests are due no later than :

User: Name .... Signature .... Date ....

Qualified Person: Name .... Signature .... Date ....

12.XLS

Reference ..../SC Page 1 of 2

STERILIZER FOR UNWRAPPED INSTRUMENTS AND UTENSILS
SUMMARY OF COMMISSIONING TEST

Hospital .... Department .... Dates(s) of tests ....

Sterilizer: Manufacturer .... Model .... Usable chamber space .... litres

Serial number .... Plant reference number ....

RESULTS OF COMMISSIONING TESTS Data file reference ....

Test (as specified in HTM 2010 * = optional)	Pass or fail	Cycle number	Start time h min s	Results
Automatic control	....	....	....	Sterilization temp (ST) selected .... °C
Instrument calibration	....	....	....	See below
Chamber temp profile	....	....	....	Max temp attained .... °C
Chamber overheat cut-out	....	....	....	Max temp attained .... °C
Thermometric small load	....	....	....	ST selected .... °C Max temp .... °C
Thermometric full load	....	....	....	ST selected .... °C Max temp .... °C
Sound pressure*	....	....		Loading area: mean ...... dBA, peak ...... dBA
				Plant room: mean ...... dBA, peak ...... dBA

Test equipment file references ....

STERILIZER INSTRUMENT CALIBRATION

Errors for instruments fitted to sterilizer as measured by test instruments during the holding time.
Sensor is *measured reading - recorded/indicated error*

	Measured	Recorder error	Indicator error
Chamber temperature	.... °C	.... °C	.... °C
Chamber pressure	.... bar	.... bar	.... bar

STERILIZER FOR UNWRAPPED INSTRUMENTS AND UTENSILS
SUMMARY OF COMMISSIONING TEST

SUMMARY OF THERMOMETRIC TESTS

Sterilization temperature (ST) selected .... °C
Automatic controller settings for plateau period: Temperature .... °C Time .... min .... s

Event	Elapsed time		Chamber pressure	Temperature sensors		
	min	s	bar	Drain/ vent °C	Load °C	Free space °C
SMALL LOAD TEST				No	No	No .....
Start of plateau period	....	....	....	....	....	....
Start of holding time	....	....	....	....	....	....
End of holding time	....	....	....	....	....	....
Maximum values attained			....	....	....	....
Equilibration time	....	....				
Holding time	....	....				
Total cycle time	....	....				
FULL LOAD TEST				No	No	No .....
Start of plateau period	....	....	....	....	....	....
Start of holding time	....	....	....	....	....	....
End of holding time	....	....	....	....	....	....
Maximum values attained			....	....	....	....
Equilibration time	....	....				
Holding time	....	....				
Total cycle time	....	....				

DECLARATION OF TEST PERSON (STERILIZERS)

1. The installation checks and tests have been completed and show that the sterilizer has been provided and installed in accordance with its specifications.
2. All test instruments have current calibration certificates.
3. Calibration of the temperature test instruments has been checked before and after the thermometric tests.
4. The commissioning tests have been completed and show that the sterilizer functions correctly when operated in accordance with operational instructions.

Test Person: Name .... Signature .... Date ....

DECLARATION OF USER
The sterilizer is fit for use. The first yearly tests are due no later than :

User: Name .... Signature .... Date ....

Reference ..../SPQ Page 1 of 2

STERILIZER FOR UNWRAPPED INSTRUMENTS AND UTENSILS
SUMMARY OF PERFORMANCE QUALIFICATION TESTS

Hospital .... Department .... Date(s) of tests ....

STERILIZER: Manufacturer .... Model .... Usable chamber space ....litres

Serial number .... Plant reference number..

Chamber shape .... Width .... mm Height ....mm Depth ....m

OPERATING CYCLE REFERENCE .... Sterilization temperature ....°C

LOADING CONDITION REFERENCE .... Batch reference ....

Nature of load ....

LOCATION OF SENSORS FOR THERMOMETRIC PQ TEST

Enter positions of temperature sensors within the chamber related to the bottom left-hand corner of a rectangular box viewed from the loading end.

Sensor number	Sensor type	Width (X) mm	Height (Y) mm	Depth (Z) mm	Location of sensor
1	T				Active chamber drain/vent
2	T				
3	T				
4	T				
5	T				
6	T				
7	T				
8	T				
9	T				
10	T				
11	T				
12	T				
13	P				Chamber pressure test port

(T = Temperature P = Pressure)

Test equipment file references ....

STERILIZER FOR UNWRAPPED INSTRUMENTS AND UTENSILS
SUMMARY OF PERFORMANCE QUALIFICATION TESTS

SUMMARY OF THERMOMETRIC PQ TEST

Sterilization temperature (ST) selected .... °C

Automatic controller setting for plateau period: Temperature .... °C Time .... min .... s

Identify sensors in the load which are the fastest and the slowest to attain the ST. Enter elapsed times and measured chamber pressures and temperatures.

Sensor number	Description	Sensor first attains ST		Sensor falls below ST		Time above ST	Max temp
		Time min s	Press bar	Time min s	Press bar	min s	°C
....	Drain/vent	....	....	....	....	....	....
....	Fastest	....	....	....	....	....	....
....	Slowest	....	....	....	....	....	....

Equilibration time ..... min ..... s Holding time ..... min ..... s Total cycle time ..... min ..... s

Cycle number .... Master Process Record reference ....

Is a microbiological PQ test required for this loading condition? ....

Result of microbiological test PASS/FAIL PQ report reference ....

DECLARATION OF TEST PERSON (STERILZERS)

1. This test has been preceded by a satisfactory sequence of commissioning/yearly tests.
   Reference ....
2. All test instruments have current calibration certificates.
3. Calibration of the thermometric test instruments has been verified before and after the thermometric tests.
4. The performance qualification tests show that the sterilizer produces acceptable product with the loading condition identified above.

Test Person: Name .... Signature .... Date ....

DECLARATION OF USER

The sterilizer is fit for use with the loading condition identified above. The first performance requalification test, due ....

User: Name .... Signature .... Date ....

Reference ..../SY   Page 1 of 1

STERILIZER FOR UNWRAPPED INSTRUMENTS AND UTENSILS
SUMMARY OF YEARLY/REVALIDATION TESTS

Hospital .... Department .... Date (s) of tests ....

STERILIZER: Manufacturer .... Model .... Usable chamber space .... litres

Serial number .... Plant reference number ....

RESULTS OF YEARLY/REVALIDATION TESTS   Data file reference ....

pecified in HTM 2010)	Pass or fail	Cycle number	Start time h min s	Results
Yearly safety checks	....			
Automatic control	....	....	....	Sterilization temp (ST) selected ..... °C
Instrument calibration	....	....	....	
Chamber overheat cut-out	....	....	....	Mac temp attained ..... °C
Thermometric small load	....	....	....	ST selected ..... °C Max temp ..... °C
Thermometric full load	....	....	....	ST selected ..... °C Max temp ..... °C

PERFORMANCE REQUALIFICATION (as required by user)

PQ report reference	Loading condition ref	Operating cycle ref	ST °C	Thermometric			Microbio. (optional)	
				Pass or fail	Cycle number	Start time h min s	Pass or fail	
....	....	....	....	....	....	....	....	
....	....	....	....	....	....	....	....	
....	....	....	....	....	....	....	....	

Test equipment file references ....

DECLARATION OF TEST PERSON (STERILIZERS) AND USER

1. All test instruments have current calibration certificates.
2. Calibration of the temperature test instruments has been checked before and after the thermometric tests.
3. The yearly/revalidation checks and tests have been completed and confirm that the sterilizer is safe to use and that commissioning and performance qualification data collected during validation remain valid.

Test Person: Name .... Signature .... Date ....

DECLARATION OF USER

The sterilizer is fit for use. The first yearly tests are due no later than :

User: Name .... Signature .... Date ....

Reference ..../SC

DRY HEAT STERILIZER - SUMMARY OF COMMISSIONING TESTS

Hospital .... Department .... Dates(s) of tests ....

Sterilizer: Manufacturer .... Model .... Usable chamber space .... litres

Serial number .... Plant reference number ....

RESULTS OF COMMISSIONING TESTS

Data file reference ....

Test (as specified in HTM 2010 * = optional)	Pass or fail	Cycle number	Start time h min s	Results
Automatic control	....	....	....	Sterilization temp (ST) selected .... °C
Instrument calibration	....	....	....	See below
Chamber temp profile	....	....	....	Max temperature.......... °C
Chamber overheat cut-out	....	....	....	Max temperature.......... °C
Basic Performance*	....	....	....	Heat-up time .... min Drift .... °C
				Overshoot.......... °C Variation .... degs C

Test equipment file references ....

STERILIZER INSTRUMENT CALIBRATION

Errors for instruments fitted to sterilizer as measured by test instruments during the holding time.
Sensor is *measured reading - recorded/indicated error*

	Measured	Recorder error	Indicator error
Chamber temperature	.... °C	.... °C	.... °C
Load Temperature (1)	.... °C	.... °C	
Load Temperature (2)	.... °C	.... °C	

DECLARATION OF TEST PERSON (STERILIZERS)

1. The installation checks and tests have been completed and show that the sterilizer has been provided and installed in accordance with its specifications.
2. All test instruments have current calibration certificates.
3. Calibration of the temperature test instruments has been checked before and after the thermometric tests.
4. The commissioning tests have been completed and show that the sterilizer functions correctly when operated in accordance with operational instructions.

Test Person: Name .... Signature .... Date ....

DECLARATION OF USER AND FOR MEDICINAL PRODUCTS QUALIFIED PERSON

The sterilizer is fit for use. The first yearly tests are due no later than :

User: Name .... Signature .... Date ....

Qualified Person: Name .... Signature .... Date ....

16.XLS

Reference ..../SPQ Page 1 of 2

DRY HEAT STERILIZER - SUMMARY OF PERFORMANCE QUALIFICATION TESTS

Hospital .... Department .... Date(s) of tests ....

STERILIZER: Manufacturer .... Model .... Usable chamber space ....litres

Serial number .... Plant reference number...

Chamber shape .... Width .... mm Height .... m Depth ....m

OPERATING CYCLE REFERENCE .... Sterilization temperature ....°C

LOADING CONDITION REFERENCE .... Batch reference ....

Nature of load ....

LOCATION OF SENSORS FOR THERMOMETRIC PQ TEST

Enter positions of temperature sensors within the chamber related to the bottom left-hand corner of a rectangular box viewed from the loading end.

Sensor number	Sensor type	Width (X) mm	Height (Y) mm	Depth (Z) mm	Location of sensor
1	T				On temperature recorder sensor
2	T				On temperature indicator sensor
3	T				
4	T				
5	T				
6	T				
7	T				
8	T				
9	T				
10	T				
11	T				
12	T				
13	P				Differential pressure across filter

(T = Temperature P = Pressure)

Test equipment file references ....

Reference ..../SPQ Page 2 of 2

DRY HEAT STERILIZER - SUMMARY OF PERFORMANCE QUALIFICATION TESTS

SUMMARY OF THERMOMETRIC PQ TEST

Sterilization temperature (ST) selected .... °C

Automatic controller setting for plateau period: Temperature .... °C Time .... min .... s

Cooling temperature setting .... °C Fo setting* .... min

Identify sensors in the load which are the fastest and the slowest to attain the ST. Enter elapsed times and measured chamber pressures and temperatures.

Sensor number	Description	Sensor first attains ST		Sensor falls below ST		Time above ST	Max temp	Fo*
		Time min s	Press bar	Time min s	Press bar	min s	°C	min
1.	Temp recorder	....	....	....	....	....	....	....
2.	Temp indicator	....	....	....	....	....	....	....
....	Fastest	....	....	....	....	....	....	....
....	Slowest	....	....	....	....	....	....	....

Equilibration time ..... min ..... s Holding time ..... min ..... s Total cycle time ..... min ..... s

Cooling stage - minimum differential pressure across air filter: ..... millbars/pascals

Temp of hottest container at end .... °C (sensor .....)

Cycle number .... Master Process Record reference ....

Is a microbiological PQ test required for this loading condition? ....

Result of microbiological test PASS/FAIL PQ report reference ....

DECLARATION OF TEST PERSON (STERILIZERS)

1. This test has been preceded by a satisfactory sequence of commissioning/yearly tests. Reference ....
2. All test instruments have current calibration certificates.
3. Calibration of the thermometric test instruments has been verified before and after the thermometric tests.
4. The performance qualification tests show that the sterilizer produces acceptable product with the loading condition identified above.

Test Person: Name .... Signature .... Date ....

DECLARATION OF USER AND FOR MEDICAL PRODUCTS QUALIFIED PERSON

The sterilizer is fit for use with the loading condition identified above. The first performance requalification test, due ....

User: Name .... Signature .... Date ....

Qualified Person: Name .... Signature .... Date ....

Reference ..../SY Page 1 of 1

DRY HEAT STERILIZER - SUMMARY OF YEARLY/REVALIDATION TESTS

Hospital .... Department .... Date (s) of tests ....

STERILIZER: Manufacturer .... Model .... Usable chamber space .... litres

Serial number .... Plant reference number ....

RESULTS OF YEARLY/REVALIDATION TESTS

Data file reference ....

pecified in HTM 2010)	Pass or fail	Cycle number	Start time h min s	Results
Yearly safety checks	....			
Automatic control	....	....	....	Sterilization temp (ST) selected ..... °C
Instrument calibration		....	....	
Chamber overheat cut-out	....	....	....	Max temp attained .... °C

PERFORMANCE REQUALIFICATION

PQ report reference	Loading condition ref	Operating cycle ref	ST °C	Thermometric			Microbio. (optional)	
				Pass or fail	Cycle number	Start time h min s	Pass or fail	
....	....	....	....	....	....	....	....	
....	....	....	....	....	....	....	....	
....	....	....	....	....	....	....	....	
....	....	....	....	....	....	....	....	
....	....	....	....	....	....	....	....	

Test equipment file references ....

DECLARATION OF TEST PERSON (STERILIZERS)

1. All test instruments have current calibration certificates.
2. Calibration of the temperature test instruments has been checked before and after the thermometric tests.
3. The yearly/revalidation checks and tests have been completed and confirm that the sterilizer is safe to use and that commissioning and performance qualification data collected during validation remain valid.

Test Person: Name .... Signature .... Date ....

DECLARATION OF USER AND FOR MEDICAL PRODUCTS QUALIFIED PERSON

The sterilizer is fit for use. The first yearly tests are due no later than :

User: Name .... Signature .... Date ....

Qualified Person: Name .... Signature .... Date ....

Reference ..../SC Page 1 of 2

LOW-TEMPERATURE STEAM DISINFECTOR
LOW-TEMPERATURE STEAM AND FORMALDEHYDE STERLIZER
SUMMARY OF COMMISSIONING TEST

Hospital .... Department .... Dates(s) of tests ....

Sterilizer: Manufacturer .... Model .... Usable chamber space .... litres

Serial number .... Plant reference number ....

RESULTS OF COMMISSIONING TESTS Data file reference ....

Test (as specified in HTM 2010 * = optional)	Pass or fail	Cycle number	Start time h min s	Results
Steam non-condensable gas	....			Concentration of NCG .... %
Steam superheat	....			Superheat .... °C
Stem dryness	....			Dryness value ....
Automatic control	....	....	....	Sterilization temp (ST) selected .... °C
Instrument calibration	....	....	....	See below
Vacuum leak monitor	....	....	....	
Chamber temp profile		....	....	Max temp attained .... °C
Chamber overheat cut-out	....	....	....	Chamber cut-out: Max temp .... °C
		....	....	Jacket cut-out: Max temp .... °C
Chamber wall temperature	....	....	....	Max temp attained .... °C
Thermometric small load	....	....	....	ST selected .... °C Max temp .... °C
Load dryness*	....	....		Average gain in mass .... %
Thermometric full load	....	....	....	ST selected .... °C Max temp .... °C
Load dryness*	....	....		Average gain in mass .... %
Basic performance	....	....	....	Holding time ..... min ..... s
Environ formaldehyde	....	....	....	Average gas concentration .... ppm
Vacuum leak (final)	....	....		Leak rate .... mbar/min
Sound pressure*	....	....		Loading area: mean ...... dBA, peak ...... dBA
				Plant room: mean ...... dBA, peak ...... dBA

Test equipment file references ....

STERILIZER INSTRUMENT CALIBRATION

Errors for instruments fitted to sterilizer as measured by test instruments during the holding time.
Sense is measured reading = recorded/indicated error

	Measured	Recorder error	Indicator error
Chamber temperature	.... °C	.... °C	.... °C
Chamber pressure	.... bar	.... bar	.... bar

Reference ..../SC   Page 2 of 2

LOW-TEMPERATURE STEAM DISINFECTOR
LOW-TEMPERATURE STEAM AND FORMALDEHYDE STERLIZER
SUMMARY OF COMMISSIONING TEST

SUMMARY OF THERMOMETRIC TESTS

Sterilization temperature (ST) selected .... °C
Automatic controller settings for plateau period: Temperature .... °C Time .... min .... s

Event	Elapsed time		Chamber pressure	Temperature sensors		
	min	s	bar	Drain/ vent °C	Test pack °C	Free space °C
SMALL LOAD TEST				No	No	No .....
Start of plateau period	....	....	....	....	....	....
Start of holding time	....	....	....	....	....	....
End of holding time	....	....	....	....	....	....
Maximum values attained			....	....	....	....
Equilibration time	....	....				
Holding time	....	....				
Total cycle time	....	....				
FULL LOAD TEST				No	No	No .....
Start of plateau period	....	....	....	....	....	....
Start of holding time	....	....	....	....	....	....
End of holding time	....	....	....	....	....	....
Maximum values attained			....	....	....	....
Equilibration time	....	....				
Holding time	....	....				
Total cycle time	....	....				

SUMMARY OF MICROBIOLOGICAL TEST FOR BASIC PERFORMANCE*

Automatic controller settings for plateau period: Temperature .... °C Time .... min .... s
Primary material .... Batch .... Expiry date ....
Primary material used in the cycle .... Setting .... millilitres Measured .... mg/litre

DECLARATION OF TEST PERSON (STERILIZERS)

1. The installation checks and tests have been completed and show that the sterilizer has been provided and installed in accordance with its specifications.
2. All test instruments have current calibration certificates.
3. Calibration of the temperature test instruments has been checked before and after the thermometric tests.
4. The commissioning tests have been completed and show that the sterilizer functions correctly when operated in accordance with operational instructions.

Test Person: Name .... Signature .... Date ....

DECLARATION OF CONSULTANT MICROBIOLOGIST

The results of the microbiologist test for basic performance are satisfactory.

Microbiologist: Name .... Signature .... Date ....

DECLARATION OF USER

The sterilizer is fit for use.The first yearly tests are due no later than: 22-Feb-95

User: Name .... Signature .... Date ....

* not required for LTS

LOW-TEMPERATURE STEAM DISINFECTOR
LOW-TEMPERATURE STEAM AND FORMALDEHYDE STERILIZER
SUMMARY OF PERFORMANCE QUALIFICATION TESTS

Hospital .... Department .... Date(s) of tests ....

STERILIZER: Manufacturer .... Model .... Usable chamber space ....litres

Serial number .... Plant reference number..

Chamber shape .... Width .... mm Height ....mm Depth ....m

OPERATING CYCLE REFERENCE .... Sterilization temperature ....°C

LOADING CONDITION REFERENCE .... Batch reference ....

Nature of load ....

LOCATION OF SENSORS FOR THERMOMETRIC PQ TEST

Enter positions of temperature sensors within the chamber related to the bottom left-hand corner of a rectangular box viewed from the loading end.

Sensor number	Sensor Type	Width (X) mm	Height (Y) mm	Depth (Z) mm	Location of sensor
1	T				Active chamber drain/vent
2	T				
3	T				
4	T				
5	T				
6	T				
7	T				
8	T				
9	T				
10	T				
11	T				
12	T				
13	P				Chamber pressure test port

(T = Temperature P = Pressure)

Test equipment file references ....

Reference ..../SPQ Page 2 of 2

LOW-TEMPERATURE STEAM DISINFECTOR
LOW-TEMPERATURE STEAM AND FORMALDEHYDE STERILIZER
SUMMARY OF PERFORMANCE QUALIFICATION TESTS

SUMMARY OF THERMOMETRIC PQ TEST

Sterilization temperature (ST) selected .... °C

Automatic controller setting for plateau period: Temperature .... °C Time .... min .... s

Identify sensors in the load which are the fastest and the slowest to attain the ST. Enter elapsed times and measured chamber pressures and temperatures.

Sensor number	Description	Sensor first attains ST		Sensor falls below ST		Time above ST	Max temp
		Time min s	Press bar	Time min s	Press bar	min s	°C
....	Drain/vent	....	....	....	....	....	....
....	Fastest	....	....	....	....	....	....
....	Slowest	....	....	....	....	....	....

Equilibration time ..... min ..... s Holding time ..... min ..... s Total cycle time ..... min ..... s

Cycle number .... Master Process Record reference ....

*RESULT OF MICROBIOLOGICAL PQ TEST: PASS/FAIL Cycle no. ....

*RESULT OF ENVIRONMENTAL GAS TEST: PASS/FAIL Cycle no. .... Average gas concentration .... ppm

DECLARATION OF TEST PERSON (STERILZERS)

1. This test has been preceded by a satisfactory sequence of commissioning/yearly tests.
   Reference ....
2. All test instruments have current calibration certificates.
3. Calibration of the thermometric test instruments has been verified before and after the thermometric tests.
4. The performance qualification tests show that the sterilizer produces acceptable product with the loading condition identified above.

Test Person: Name .... Signature .... Date ....

DECLARATION OF CONSULTANT MICROBIOLOGIST
The results of the microbiological test for performance qualification are satisfactory.

Microbiologist: Name .... Signature .... Date ....

DECLARATION OF USER

The sterilizer is fit for use with the loading condition identified above. The first performance requalification test, due ....

User: Name .... Signature .... Date ....

* not required for LTS

Reference ..../SY   Page 1 of 1

LOW-TEMPERATURE STEAM DISINFECTOR
LOW-TEMPERATURE STEAM AND FORMALDEHYDE STERILIZER
SUMMARY OF YEARLY/REVALIDATION TESTS

Hospital .... Department .... Date (s) of tests ....

STERILIZER: Manufacturer .... Model .... Usable chamber space .... litres

Serial number .... Plant reference number ....

RESULTS OF YEARLY/REVALIDATION TESTS   Data file reference ....

Test (as specified in HTM 2010)	Pass or fail	Cycle number	Start time h min s	Results
Yearly safety checks	....			
Chamber overheat cut-out	....	....	....	Max temp attained ..... °C
Chamber wall temperature	....	....	....	Max temp attained ..... °C
Automatic control	....	....	....	Sterilization temp (ST) selected ..... °C
Instrument calibration	....	....	....	
Vacuum leak monitor	....	....	....	
Thermometric small load	....	....	....	ST selected ..... °C Max temp ..... °C
Thermometric full load	....	....	....	ST selected ..... °C Max temp ..... °C
Basic performance	....	....	....	
Environment formaldehyde	....	....	....	Average gas concentration ..... ppm
Vacuum leak (final)	....	....	....	Leak rate .... mbar/min

PERFORMANCE REQUALIFICATION (if required)

PQ report reference	Loading condition ref	Operating cycle ref	ST °C	Thermometric			Microbio	Env. gas
				Pass or fail	Cycle number	Start time h min s	Pass or fail	Pass or fail
....	....	....	....	....	....	....	....	....
....	....	....	....	....	....	....	....	....
....	....	....	....	....	....	....	....	....

Test equipment file references ....

DECLARATION OF TEST PERSON (STERILIZERS) AND USER

1. All test instruments have current calibration certificates.
2. Calibration of the temperature test instruments has been checked before and after the thermometric tests.
3. The yearly/revalidation checks and tests have been completed and confirm the sterilizer is safe to use and the commissioning and performance qualification data collected during validation remain valid.

Test Person: Name .... Signature .... Date ....

DECLARATION OF MICROBIOLOGIST
The results of the microbiological test are satisfactory.

Microbiologist: Name .... Signature .... Date ....

DECLARATION OF USER
The sterilizer is fit for use. The first yearly tests are due no later than :

User: Name .... Signature .... Date ....

* not required for LTS

6.XLS

LOW-TEMPERATURE STEAM AND FORMALDEHYDE STERILIZER
REPORT OF MICROBIOLOGICAL AND CHEMICAL INDICATOR TEST FOR BASIC PERFORMANCE

utomatic controller settings for plateau period: Temperature_________°C Time____min____sec's

rimary materials for generating formaldehyde Batch No_____________Expiry Date___________

Manufacture _______________________ Reference Certificate No ___________

Batch No __________Expiry Date _________Chemical Indicator Batch No ___________Expiry Date ________

Mass of primary material use in cycle Setting ______gram Measured _______gram

Biological Indicators (BI) Organism _______________________________ Strain _____________

Manufactures declared number of recoverable spores on each indicator __________________Expiry Date ________

Batch No ______________ Process Cycle Number____________________Date_________________

EST PERSON
Name...Signature...Date................................

Location of Chemical and Biological Indicators

Location	No	Biological Chemical	No	Biological Chemical	No	Biological Chemical
Rear plane	1	Pass/Fail Pass/Fail	2	Pass/Fail Pass/Fail	3	Pass/Fail Pass/Fail
	4	Pass/Fail Pass/Fail	5	Pass/Fail Pass/Fail	6	Pass/Fail Pass/Fail
	7	Pass/Fail Pass/Fail	8	Pass/Fail Pass/Fail	9	Pass/Fail Pass/Fail
Centre plane	10	Pass/Fail Pass/Fail	11	Pass/Fail Pass/Fail	12	Pass/Fail Pass/Fail
	13	Pass/Fail Pass/Fail	14	Pass/Fail Pass/Fail	15	Pass/Fail Pass/Fail
	16	Pass/Fail Pass/Fail	17	Pass/Fail Pass/Fail	18	Pass/Fail Pass/Fail
Front plane	19	Pass/Fail Pass/Fail	20	Pass/Fail Pass/Fail	21	Pass/Fail Pass/Fail
	22	Pass/Fail Pass/Fail	23	Pass/Fail Pass/Fail	24	Pass/Fail Pass/Fail
	25	Pass/Fail Pass/Fail	26	Pass/Fail Pass/Fail	27	Pass/Fail Pass/Fail

Line Pickerall Helices	Wrapped	No1	Pass/Fail Pass/Fail	No2	Pass/Fail Pass/Fail
	Unwrapped	No3	Pass/Fail Pass/Fail	No4	Pass/Fail Pass/Fail

Biological Controls

Unexposed BI	No1	Growth/No growth	No2	Growth/No growth	No3	Growth/No growth
No BI	No4	Growth/No growth	No5	Growth/No growth	No6	Growth/No growth

Test performed by:- NAME...Signature....................................Date............................

NAME...Signature....................................Date............................

NAME...Signature....................................Date............................

DoH 5c5

ETHYLENE OXIDE STERILIZER - SUMMARY OF COMMISSIONING TESTS

Hospital .... Department .... Date(s) of tests ....

STERILISER: Manufacturer .... Model .... Usable chamber space .... litres

Serial number .... Plant reference number ....

Composition of gas .... Gas source .... Preset gas exposure temperature ....°C

RESULTS OF COMMISSIONING TESTS

Data file reference ....

Test (as specified in HTM 2010 * = optional)	Pass or fail	Cycle number	Start time h min s	Results
Pressure leak*	....	....		Leak rate ....mbar/min
Automatic control	....	....	....	
Instrument calibration	....	....	....	See below
Vacuum leak monitor	....	....	....	
Chamber temp profile	....	....	....	
Chamber overheat cut-out	....	....	....	Chamber cut-out: Max temp ....°C
	....	....	....	Jacket cut-out: Max temp ....°C
Chamber wall temperature	....	....	....	Max temp attained ....°C
Chamber space temperature	....	....	....	Max temp attained ....°C
Gas circulation*	....	....	....	
Gas exposure time	....	....	....	Critical GET .... h .... min .... s
Vacuum leak (final)	....	....		Leak rate .... mbar/min
Sound pressure*	....	....		Loading area: mean .... dBA, peak .... dBA
				Plant room: mean .... dBA, peak .... dBA

Test equipment file references ....

STERILIZER INSTRUMENT CALIBRATION

Errors for instruments fitted to sterilizer as measured by test instruments during the holding time.

Sensor is *measured reading - recorded/indicated error*

	Measured	Recorder error	Indicator error
Chamber temperature	..........................°C	..........................°C	..........................°C
Jacket temperature	..........................°C	..........................°C	..........................°C
Chamber pressure	.... bar	.... bar	.... bar
Chamber humidity	.... %RH	.... %RH	.... %RH

* If applicable

Reference .... /SC   Page 2 of 2

SUMMARY OF MICROBIOLOGICAL TEST FOR GAS EXPOSURE TIME (GET)

Jacket overheat cut-out setting .... °C
Chamber overheat cut-out setting ....°C

Vacuum leak monitor setting .... mbar
Pressure leak monitor setting .... mbar

Cycle no	Gas exposure time h min s	No. BIs surviving
....	....	....
....	....	....
....	....	....
....	....	....
....	....	....
....	....	....

Critical GET (shortest with no survivors)
.... h .... min .... s

Recommended GET for production loads
.... h .... min .... s

SET AND DETERMINE VALUES OF CYCLE VARIABLES FOR CRITICAL GAS EXPOSURE TIME

Cycle variable	Set value	Determined	Method of determination
Mass of gas used	.... g	.... g	....
EO concentration	.... g/1	.... g/1	....
Minimum chamber temperature	.... °C	.... °C	....
Minimum chamber pressure	.... bar	.... bar	....
Maximum chamber pressure	.... bar	.... bar	....
Minimum chamber humidity	.... %RH	.... %RH	....

DECLARATION OF TEST PERSON (STERILIZERS)

1. The installation checks and tests have been completed and show that the sterilizer has been provided and installed in accordance with its specifications.
2. All test instruments have current calibration certificates.
3. Calibration of the temperature test instruments has been checked before and after the thermometric tests.
4. The commissioning tests have been completed and show that the sterilizer functions correctly when operated in accordance with operational instructions.

Test Person: Name .... Signature .... Date ....

DECLARATION OF CONSULTANT MICROBIOLOGIST

The results of the microbiological test for gas exposure time are satisfactory.

Microbiologist: Name .... Signature .... Date ....

DECLARATION OF USER

The steriliser is fit for use. The first yearly tests are due no later than ....

User: Name .... Signature .... Date ....

Reference .... /SPQ Page 1 of 2

ETHYLENE OXIDE STERILIZER - SUMMARY OF PERFORMANCE QUALIFICATION TESTS

Hospital .... Department .... Date(s) of tests ....

STERILIZER: Manufacturer .... Model .... Usable chamber space .... litre

Serial number .... Plant reference number ....

Composition of gas .... Gas source .... Preset gas exposure temperature ....°C

Chamber shape .... Width ....mm Height ....mm Depth ....mm

OPERATING CYCLE: Mass of gas .... g Gas exposure time ..... h ..... min ..... s

LOADING CONDITION REFERENCE .... Batch reference ....

Nature of load ....

LOCATION OF SENSORS FOR PARAMETRIC PQ TEST

Enter positions of sensors within the chamber related to the bottom left-hand corner of a rectangular box viewed from the loading end.

Sensor number	Type	Width (X) mm	Height (Y) mm	Depth (Z) mm	Location of sensor
....	....	....	....	....	On temperature recorder sensor
....	....	....	....	....	Gas entry port*
....	....	....	....	....	Gas preheater*
....	....	....	....	....	....
....	....	....	....	....	....
....	....	....	....	....	....
....	....	....	....	....	....
....	....	....	....	....	....
....	....	....	....	....	....
....	....	....	....	....	....
....	....	....	....	....	....
....	....	....	....	....	....
....	....	....	....	....	....
....	....	....	....	....	Chamber pressure port
....	....	....	....	....	Chamber free space
....	....	....	....	....	Load

(T = temperature RH = relative humidity P = pressure)

Test equipment file references ....

Reference .... /SPQ Page 2 of 2

ETHYLENE OXIDE STERILIZER - SUMMARY OF PERFORMANCE QUALIFICATION TESTS

SUMMARY OF PARAMETRIC PQ TEST

Sterilization temperature (ST) .... °C

Automatic controller settings for plateau period: Temperature ....°C Time .... min .... s

Identify sensors in the load which are the fastest and the slowest to attain the ST. Enter elapsed times and measured chamber pressures and temperatures.

Humidity and temperature in chamber at the end of conditioning period ....%RH ....°C

Humidity and temperature in the load if in hottest part of chamber ....%RH ....°C

Sensor number	Description	Sensor first attains ST		Sensor fails below ST		Time above ST	Max temp
		Time min s	Press bar	Time min s	Press bar	min s	°C
1.	Recorder sensor	....	....	....	....	....	....
2.*	Gas entry port	....	....	....	....	....	....
3.*	Gas preheater	....	....	....	....	....	....
.....	Slowest load item	....	....	....	....	....	....
.....	Hottest surface	....	....	....	....	....	....
.....	Coolest surface	....	....	....	....	....	....
.....	Coolest space	....	....	....	....	....	....

Equilibration time .....min .....s Holding time .....min .....s Total cycle time .....min .....s

Cycle number .... Master Process Record reference ....

RESULT OF MICROBIOLOGICAL PQ TEST PASS / FAIL

RESULT OF ENVIRONMENTAL GAS TEST PASS / FAIL Average gas concentration .... ppm

DECLARATION OF TEST PERSON (STERILIZERS)

1. This test has been preceded by a satisfactory sequence of commissioning/yearly tests. Reference ....
2. All test instruments have current calibration certificates.
3. Calibration of the thermometric test instruments has been verified before and after the thermometric tests.
4. The performance qualification tests show that the sterilizer produces acceptable product with the loading conditio identified above.

Test Person: Name .... Signature .... Date ....

DECLARATION OF CONSULTANT MICROBIOLOGIST

The results of the microbiological test for performance qualification are satisfactory.

Microbiologist: Name .... Signature .... Date ....

DECLARATION OF USER

The sterilizer is fit for use with the loading condition identified above. The first performance requalification test, due ....

User: Name .... Signature .... Date ....

* not required on cartridge systems

Reference ..../SY Page 1 of 1

ETHYLENE OXIDE STERILIZER - SUMMARY OF YEARLY/REVALIDATION TESTS

Hospital .... Department .... Dates (s) of tests ....
Sterilizer: Manufacturer .... Model .... Usable chamber space .... litre
Serial number .... Plant reference number ....
Composition of gas .... Gas source .... Preset gas exposure temperature ....°C

RESULTS OF YEARLY/REVALIDATION TESTS Data file reference ....

Test (as specified in HTM 2010)	Pass or fail	Cycle number	Start time h min s	Results
Yearly safety checks	....			
Pressure leak*	....	....		Leak rate .... mbar/min
Automatic control	....	....	....	
Instrument calibration	....	....	....	See below
Chamber temp profile	....	....	....	
Chamber overheat cut-out	....	....	....	Chamber cut-out: Max temp ....°C
		....	....	Jacket cut-out: Max temp ....°C
Chamber wall temperature	....	....	....	Max temp attained ....°C
Chamber space temperature	....	....	....	Max temp attained ....°C
Gas circulation*	....	....	....	
Basic performance	....	....	....	Critical GET ..... h ..... min .....s
Vacuum leak (final)	....	....		Leak rate .... mbar/min
Vacuum leak monitor	....	....		

PERFORMANCE REQUALIFICATION

PQ report reference	Loading Conditional ref	Operating Cycle ref	ST °C	Thermometric			Microbio	Env. gas
				Pass or fail	Cycle number	Start time h min s	Pass or fail	Pass or fail
....	....	....	....	....	....	....	....	....
....	....	....	....	....	....	....	....	....
....	....	....	....	....	....	....	....	....

Test equipment reference ....

DECLARATION OF TEST PERSON (STERILIZERS)

1. All test instruments have current calibration certificates.
2. Calibration of the temperature test instruments has been checked before and after the thermometric tests.
3. The yearly/revalidation checks and tests have been completed and confirm that the sterlizer is safe to use and that commissioning and performance qualification data collected during validation remain valid.

Test Person: Name .... Signature .... Date ....

DECLARATION OF MICROBIOLOGIST

The results of the microbiological test are satisfactory.

Microbiologist: Name .... Signature .... Date ....

DECLARATION OF USER

The sterilizer is fit for use. The first yearly tests are due no later than :

User: Name .... Signature .... Date ....

* if applicable

3.XLS

ETHYLENE OXIDE STERILIZER
REPORT OF MICROBIOLOGICAL TEST FOR BASIC PERFORMANCE

Automatic controller settings for plateau period: Temperature_________°C Time____min____sec's

Pre-set gas exposure Temperature _______°C Composition of gas________________Gas source _________

Manufacture ________________________ Reference Certificate No ____________

Batch No ___________Expiry Date __________Chemical Indicator Batch No ___________Expiry Date _________

Mass of primary material use in cycle Setting ______gram Measured _______gram

Biological Indicators (BI) Organism ______________________________Strain ____________________

Manufactures declared number of recoverable spores on each indicator ___________________Expiry Date _________

Batch No _______________ Process Cycle Number___________________Date__________________

TEST PERSON
Name..Signature...Date..

Location of Chemical and Biological Indicators

Location	No	Biological	Chemical	No	Biological	Chemical	No	Biological	Chemical
Rear plane	1	Pass/Fail	Pass/Fail	2	Pass/Fail	Pass/Fail	3	Pass/Fail	Pass/Fail
	4	Pass/Fail	Pass/Fail	5	Pass/Fail	Pass/Fail	6	Pass/Fail	Pass/Fail
	7	Pass/Fail	Pass/Fail	8	Pass/Fail	Pass/Fail	9	Pass/Fail	Pass/Fail
Centre plane	10	Pass/Fail	Pass/Fail	11	Pass/Fail	Pass/Fail	12	Pass/Fail	Pass/Fail
	13	Pass/Fail	Pass/Fail	14	Pass/Fail	Pass/Fail	15	Pass/Fail	Pass/Fail
	16	Pass/Fail	Pass/Fail	17	Pass/Fail	Pass/Fail	18	Pass/Fail	Pass/Fail
Front plane	19	Pass/Fail	Pass/Fail	20	Pass/Fail	Pass/Fail	21	Pass/Fail	Pass/Fail
	22	Pass/Fail	Pass/Fail	23	Pass/Fail	Pass/Fail	24	Pass/Fail	Pass/Fail
	25	Pass/Fail	Pass/Fail	26	Pass/Fail	Pass/Fail	27	Pass/Fail	Pass/Fail

Biological Controls

Unexposed BI	No1	Growth/No growth	No2	Growth/No growth	No3	Growth/No growth
No BI	No4	Growth/No growth	No5	Growth/No growth	No6	Growth/No growth

Test performed by:- NAME...Signature....................................Date............................

NAME...Signature....................................Date............................

NAME...Signature....................................Date............................

DoH 1c1

LABORATORY STERILIZER - SUMMARY OF COMMISSIONING TESTS

NAME OF PROCESS CYCLE ....

Hospital .... Department .... Dates(s) of tests ....

Sterilizer: Manufacturer .... Model .... Usable chamber space .... litres

Serial number .... Plant reference number ....

RESULTS OF COMMISSIONING TESTS

Data file reference ....

Test (as specified in HTM 2010 * = Optional)	Pass or fail	Cycle number	Start time h min s	Results/notes
Automatic control	....	....	....	Sterilization temp (ST) selected .... °C
Instrument calibration	....	....	....	See below
Chamber temp profile	....	....	....	Max temperature attained .... °C
Thermometric small load	....	....	....	ST selected .... °C Max temp .... °C
Thermometric full load	....	....	....	ST selected .... °C Max temp .... °C
Vacuum leak (final)**	....	....		Leak rate .... mbar/min
Thermal door-lock**	....	....		
Sound pressure*	....	....		Loading area: mean ..... dBA, peak ..... dBA
				Plant area: mean ..... dBA, peak ..... dBA

Test equipment file references ....

STERILIZER INSTRUMENT CALIBRATION

Errors for instruments fitted to sterilizer as measured by test instruments during the holding time.
Sense is measured reading = recorded/indicated error

	Measured	Recorder error	Indicator error
Chamber temperature	.... °C	.... °C	.... °C
Load temperature (1)**	.... °C	.... °C	.... °C**
Load temperature (2)**	.... °C	.... °C	.... °C**
Chamber pressure	.... bar	.... bar	.... bar

** if applicable

Reference ..../SC Page 2 of 2

LABORATORY STERILIZER - SUMMARY OF COMMISSIONING TESTS

NAME OF PROCESS CYCLE ....

SUMMARY OF THERMOMETRIC TESTS

Sterilization temperature (ST) selected .... °C
Automatic controller settings for plateau period: Temperature .... °C Time .... min .... s
Door release temperature setting .... °C Fo Setting .... min*

Event	Elapsed time		Chamber pressure	Temperature sensors		
				Drain/ vent °C	Fast °C	Slow °C
	min	s	bar			
SMALL LOAD TEST				No	No	No .....
Start of plateau period	....	....	....	....	....	....
Start of holding time	....	....	....	....	....	....
End of holding time	....	....	....	....	....	....
Maximum values attained			....	....	....	....
Fo value at end*				..... min	..... min	..... min
Equilibration time	....	....				
Holding time	....	....				
Total cycle time	....	....				

Temperature of hottest load item when cycle complete .... °C (sensor no. .....)

Event	min	s	bar	Drain/ vent °C	Fast °C	Slow °C
FULL LOAD TEST				No	No	No .....
Start of plateau period	....	....	....	....	....	....
Start of holding time	....	....	....	....	....	....
End of holding time	....	....	....	....	....	....
Maximum values attained			....	....	....	....
Fo value at end*				..... min	..... min	..... min
Equilibration time	....	....				
Holding time	....	....				
Total cycle time	....	....				

Temperature of hottest load item when cycle complete .... °C (sensor no. .....)

DECLARATION OF TEST PERSON (STERILIZERS)

1. The installation checks and tests have been completed and show that the sterilizer has been provided and installed in accordance with its specifications.
2. All test instruments have current calibration certificates. Calibration of the temperature test instruments has been checked before and after the thermometric tests.
3. The commisioning tests have been completed and show that the sterilizer functions correctly on this process cycle when operated in accordance with operational instructions.

Test Person: Name .... Signature .... Date ....

DECLARATION OF USER

The sterilizer is fit for use. The first yearly tests are due no later than :

User: Name .... Signature .... Date ....

* if applicable

Reference ..../SPQ Page 1 of 2

LABORATORY STERILIZER - SUMMARY OF PERFORMANCE QUALIFICATION TESTS

NAME OF PROCESS CYCLE ....

Site .... Department .... Date(s) of tests ....

STERILIZER: Manufacturer .... Model .... Usable chamber space ....litres

Serial number .... Plant reference number...

Chamber shape .... Width .... mm Height ....mm Depth ....mm

OPERATING CYCLE REFERENCE .... Sterilization temperature ....°C

LOADING CONDITION REFERENCE ....

Nature of load ....

LOCATION OF SENSORS FOR THERMOMETRIC PQ TEST

Enter positions of temperature sensors within the chamber related to the bottom left-hand corner of a rectangular box viewed from the loading end.

Sensor number	Sensor type	Width (X) mm	Height (Y) mm	Depth (Z) mm	Location of sensor
1	T				Active chamber drain/vent
2	T				
3	T				
4	T				
5	T				
6	T				
7	T				
8	T				
9	T				
10	T				
11	T				
12	T				
13	P				Chamber pressure test port
14	P				Spray pressure test port

(T = Temperature P = Pressure)

Test equipment file references ....

Reference ..../SPQ Page 2 of 2

LABORATORY STERILIZER - SUMMARY OF PERFORMANCE QUALIFICATION TESTS

SUMMARY OF THERMOMETRIC PQ TEST

Sterilization temperature (ST) selected .... °C

Automatic controller setting for plateau period: Temperature .... °C Time .... min .... s

Door release temperature setting .... °C F. setting .... min

Identify sensors in the load which are the fastest and the slowest to attain the ST. Enter elapsed times and measured chamber pressures and temperatures.

Sensor number	Description	Sensor first attains ST		Sensor falls below ST		Time above ST	Max temp	Fo
		Time min s	Press bar	Time min s	Press bar	min s	°C	min
....	Drain/vent	....	....	....	....	....	....	....
....	Fastest	....	....	....	....	....	....	....
....	Slowest	....	....	....	....	....	....	....

Equilibration time ..... min ..... s Holding time ..... min ..... s Total cycle time ..... min ..... s

Temp of hottest load item at end .... °C (sensor .....)

Cycle number .... Master Process Record reference ....

Is a microbiological PQ test required for this loading condition? ....

Result of microbiological test PASS/FAIL PQ report reference ....

DECLARATION OF TEST PERSON (STERILIZERS)

1. This test has been preceded by a satisfactory sequence of commissioning/yearly tests. Reference ....
2. All test instruments have current calibration certificates.
3. Calibration of the thermometric test instruments has been verified before and after the thermometric tests.
4. The performance qualification tests show that the sterilizer produces acceptable product with the loading condition identified above.

Test Person: Name .... Signature .... Date ....

DECLARATION OF USER

The sterilizer is fit for use with the loading condition identified above. The first performance requalification test, due ....

User: Name .... Signature .... Date ....

Reference ..../SY Page 1 of 2

LABORATORY STERILIZER - SUMMARY OF YEARLY/REVALIDATION TESTS

Hospital .... Department .... Date (s) of tests ....

STERILIZER: Manufacturer .... Model .... Usable chamber space .... litres

Serial number .... Plant reference number ....

RESULTS OF YEARLY/REVALIDATION TESTS Data file reference ....

Test (as specified in HTM 2010) (as applicable)	Pass or fail	Cycle number	Start time h min s	Results/notes
Yearly safety checks	....			
Automatic control				
Instrument calibration	....	....	....	
Small discard	....	....	....	Sterilization temp selected .... °C
Large discard	....	....	....	Sterilization temp selected .... °C
Culture media (preset)	....	....	....	Sterilization temp selected .... °C
Culture media (variable)	....	....	....	Sterilization temp selected .... °C
Fabrics	....	....	....	Sterilization temp selected .... °C
Empty glassware	....	....	....	Sterilization temp selected .... °C
Free steaming	....	....	....	Sterilization temp selected .... °C
Thermometric small load				
Small discard	....	....	....	Sterilization temp selected .... °C
Large discard	....	....	....	Sterilization temp selected .... °C
Culture media (preset)	....	....	....	Sterilization temp selected .... °C
Culture media (variable)	....	....	....	Sterilization temp selected .... °C
Fabrics	....	....	....	Sterilization temp selected .... °C
Empty glassware	....	....	....	Sterilization temp selected .... °C
Free steaming	....	....	....	Sterilization temp selected .... °C
Thermometric full load				
Small discard	....	....	....	Sterilization temp selected .... °C
Large Discard	....	....	....	Sterilization temp selected .... °C
Culture media (preset)	....	....	....	Sterilization temp selected .... °C
Culture media (variable)	....	....	....	Sterilization temp selected .... °C
Fabrics	....	....	....	Sterilization temp selected .... °C
Empty glassware	....	....	....	Sterilization temp selected .... °C
Free steaming	....	....	....	Sterilization temp selected .... °C
Media preparator	....	....	....	Preset temp .... °C
Reheat and dispensing	....	....		
Vacuum leak test (final)	....	....		Leak rate .... mbar/min
Thermal door-lock	....	....		Setting .... °C

53.XLS

Reference ..../SY Page 2 of 2

LABORATORY STERILIZER - YEARLY/REVALIDATION

PERFORMANCE REQUALIFICATION

PQ report reference	Loading condition ref	Operating cycle ref	ST °C	Thermometric			Microbio.	Notes
				Pass or fail	Cycle number	Start time h min s	Pass or fail	
....	....	....	....	....	....	....	....	....
....	....	....	....	....	....	....	....	....
....	....	....	....	....	....	....	....	....
....	....	....	....	....	....	....	....	....
....	....	....	....	....	....	....	....	....
....	....	....	....	....	....	....	....	....
....	....	....	....	....	....	....	....	....
....	....	....	....	....	....	....	....	....
....	....	....	....	....	....	....	....	....
....	....	....	....	....	....	....	....	....
....	....	....	....	....	....	....	....	....
....	....	....	....	....	....	....	....	....
....	....	....	....	....	....	....	....	....
....	....	....	....	....	....	....	....	....
....	....	....	....	....	....	....	....	....
....	....	....	....	....	....	....	....	....

Test equipment file references ....

DECLARATION OF TEST PERSON (STERILIZERS)

1. All test instruments have current calibration certificates. Calibration of the temperature test instruments has been checked before and after the thermometric tests.
2. The yearly/revalidation checks and tests have been completed and confirm the sterilizer is safe to use and the commissioning and performance qualification data collected during validation remain valid.

Test Person: Name .... Signature .... Date ....

DECLARATION OF USER

The sterilizer is fit for use. The first yearly tests are due no later than :

User: Name .... Signature .... Date ....

Other publications in this series

(Given below are details of all Health Technical Memoranda available from HMSO. HTMs marked (*) are currently being revised, those marked (†) are out of print. Some HTMs in preparation at the time of publication of this HTM are also listed.)

- 1 Anti-static precautions: rubber, plastics and fabrics*†
- 2 Anti-static precautions: flooring in anaesthetising areas (and data processing rooms)*, 1977.
- 3 –
- 4 –
- 5 Steam boiler plant Instrumentation†
- 6 Protection of condensate systems: filming amines†
- 2007 Electrical services: supply and distribution, 1993.
- 8 –
- 9 –
- 2011 Emergency electrical services, 1993.
- 12 –
- 13 –
- 2014 Abatement of electrical interference, 1993.
- 2015 Bedhead services, 1994.
- 16 –
- 17 Health building engineering installations: commissioning and associated activities, 1978.
- 18 Facsimile telegraphy: possible applications in DGHs†
- 19 Facsimile telegraphy: the transmission of pathology reports within a hospital – a case study†
- 2020 Electrical safety code for low voltage systems, 1993.
- 2021 Electrical safety code for high voltage systems, 1993.
- 2022 Medical gas pipeline systems, 1994.
- 23 Access and accommodation for engineering services†
- 24 –
- 2025 Ventilation in healthcare premises, 1994.
- 26 Commissioning of oil, gas and dual fired boilers: with notes on design, operation and maintenance†
- 27 Cold water supply storage and mains distribution* [Revised version will deal with water storage and distribution], 1978.
- 28 to 39 –
- 2040 The control of legionellae in healthcare premises – a code of practice, 1993.
- 41 to 49 –
- 2050 Risk management in the NHS estate, 1994.
- 51 to 54 –
- 2055 Telecommunications (telephone exchanges), 1994.

Component Data Base (HTMs 54 to 70)

- 54.1 User manual, 1993.
- 55 Windows, 1989.
- 56 Partitions, 1989.
- 57 Internal glazing, 1989.
- 58 Internal doorsets, 1989.
- 59 Ironmongery, 1989.
- 60 Ceilings, 1989.
- 61 Flooring, 1989.
- 62 Demountable storage systems, 1989.
- 63 Fitted storage systems, 1989.
- 64 Sanitary assemblies, 1989.
- 65 Signs†
- 66 Cubicle curtain track, 1989.
- 67 Laboratory fitting-out system, 1993.
- 68 Ducts and panel assemblies, 1993.
- 69 Protection, 1993.
- 70 Fixings, 1993.
- 71 to 80 –

Firecode

- 81 Firecode: fire precautions in new hospitals, 1987.
- 81 Supp 1 1993.
- 82 Firecode: alarm and detection systems, 1989.
- 83 Fire safety in healthcare premises: general fire precautions, 1994.
- 85 Firecode: fire precautions in existing hospitals, 1994.
- 86 Firecode: fire risk assessment in hospitals, 1994.
- 87 Firecode: textiles and furniture, 1993.
- 88 Fire safety in health care premises: guide to fire precautions in NHS housing in the community for mentally handicapped/ill people, 1986.

New HTMs in preparation

Lifts
Washers for sterile production

Health Technical Memoranda published by HMSO can be purchased from HMSO bookshops in London (post orders to PO Box 276, SW8 5DT), Edinburgh, Belfast, Manchester, Birmingham and Bristol, or through good booksellers. HMSO provide a copy service for publications which are out of print; and a standing order service.

Enquiries about Health Technical Memoranda (but not orders) should be addressed to: NHS Estates, Department of Health, Marketing and Publications Unit, 1 Trevelyan Square, Boar Lane, Leeds LS1 6AE.

About NHS Estates

NHS Estates is an Executive Agency of the Department of Health and is involved with all aspects of health estate management, development and maintenance. The Agency has a dynamic fund of knowledge which it has acquired during 30 years of working in the field. Using this knowledge NHS Estates has developed products which are unique in range and depth. These are described below.

NHS Estates also makes its experience available to the field through its consultancy services.

Enquiries should be addressed to: NHS Estates, 1 Trevelyan Square, Boar Lane, Leeds LS1 6AE. Tel: 0532 547000.

Some other NHS Estates products

Activity DataBase – a computerised system for defining the activities which have to be accommodated in spaces within health buildings. *NHS Estates*

Design Guides – complementary to Health Building Notes, Design Guides provide advice for planners and designers about subjects not appropriate to the Health Building Notes series. *HMSO*

Estatecode – user manual for managing a health estate. Includes a recommended methodology for property appraisal and provides a basis for integration of the estate into corporate business planning. *HMSO*

Capricode – a framework for the efficient management of capital projects from inception to completion. *HMSO*

Concode – outlines proven methods of selecting contracts and commissioning consultants. Reflects official policy on contract procedures. *HMSO*

Works Information Management System – a computerised information system for estate management tasks, enabling tangible assets to be put into the context of servicing requirements. *NHS Estates*

Health Building Notes – advice for project teams procuring new buildings and adapting or extending existing buildings. *HMSO*

Health Facilities Notes – debate current and topical issues of concern across all areas of healthcare provision. *HMSO*

Health Guidance Notes – an occasional series of publications which respond to changes in Department of Health policy or reflect changing NHS operational management. Each deals with a specific topic and is complementary to a related Health Technical Memorandum. *HMSO*

Encode – shows how to plan and implement a policy of energy efficiency in a building. *HMSO*

Firecode – for policy, technical guidance and specialist aspects of fire precautions. *HMSO*

Concise – software support for managing the capital programme. Compatible with Capricode. *NHS Estates*

Model Engineering Specifications – comprehensive advice used in briefing consultants, contractors and suppliers of healthcare engineering services to meet Departmental policy and best practice guidance. *NHS Estates*

Items noted "HMSO" can be purchased from HMSO Bookshops in London (post orders to PO Box 276, SW8 5DT), Edinburgh, Belfast, Manchester, Birmingham and Bristol or through good booksellers.

Enquiries about NHS Estates should be addressed to: NHS Estates, Marketing and Publications Unit, Department of Health, 1 Trevelyan Square, Boar Lane, Leeds LS1 6AE.

NHS Estates consultancy service

Designed to meet a range of needs from advice on the oversight of estates management functions to a much fuller collaboration for particularly innovative or exemplary projects.

Enquiries should be addressed to: NHS Estates, Consultancy Service (address as above).

Printed in the United Kingdom for HMSO
Dd296842 3/94 C15 G3396 10170